LIPOSUCTION

*A Question-and-Answer Guide to
Today's Popular Cosmetic Procedure*

LIPOSUCTION

A Question-and-Answer
Guide to Today's Popular
Cosmetic Procedure

Ron M. Shelton, M.D.,
and Terry Malloy

BERKLEY BOOKS, NEW YORK

LIPOSUCTION

A Berkley Book/published by arrangement with the author

PRINTING HISTORY
Berkley mass-market edition/January 2004

Copyright © 2004 by Terry Malloy
Text design by Kristin del Rosario
Cover design by Rita Frangie
Cover photograph of woman's abdomen by Jeff Maloney, Photodisc Green, copyright © 2003.
Cover photograph of woman's legs with feet pointed by Digital Vision, The Body Collection, copyright © 2003.

For information address: The Berkley Publishing Group,
a division of Penguin Group (USA) Inc.,
375 Hudson Street, New York, New York 10014.

ISBN: 0-425-19385-3

BERKLEY®
Berkley Books are published by The Berkley Publishing Group,
a division of Penguin Group (USA) Inc.,
375 Hudson Street, New York, New York 10014.
BERKLEY and the "B" design
are trademarks belonging to Penguin Group (USA) Inc.

PRINTED IN THE UNITED STATES OF AMERICA

10 9 8 7 6 5 4 3 2 1

Ron Shelton dedicates this book to his parents, Rita and Norman, whose love, devotion, personal sacrifices, and unfailing support enabled him to realize his dream of becoming a doctor. He hopes that the care and concern they have always shown toward others is reflected in his own approach to his patients and all the others who touch his life.

Terry Malloy dedicates this book to Esther Oduh Nwajei, whose integrity and dedication to caring for others is a true inspiration.

Contents

Introduction

YOUR diet is healthy, you exercise regularly, you have a great wardrobe, and you always try to look your best. You love your job, feel close to family and friends, and enjoy many different activities. In short, your life is pretty good.

And yet, something is missing. For years, you've worked hard to make yourself as attractive and youthful as possible, but when you look in the mirror, you're still not happy.

Maybe it's those pesky bulges on your hips that you've tried to exercise away but which just won't move. Or those lumps on your inner thighs that are just like your mother's. It could be the sagging skin under your chin that keeps dragging down your face. Or perhaps it's your tummy that won't get flat no matter how many sit-ups you do every morning.

The fact is that many of us—women and men both—have unsightly fat deposits that no amount of dieting and exercise will remove. We can follow the strictest diet and work out for hours at the gym, but we always seem to lose weight in the wrong places—never where we want.

If this sounds like you, then it's very possible that you are a good candidate for what has become the most popular cosmetic surgical procedure today: liposuction.

By now, everyone has heard about liposuction and many of us have even seen it demonstrated on television. So it's entirely possible that you think you know all about it. "It's that operation where they suck out all your fat," you say, not realizing that it's a lot more complicated than that.

The truth is, most people don't really know very much about liposuction. Before you can decide if liposuction is a good way to help you lose unwanted fat, there's a great deal you should know. It is our hope that this book will be a comprehensive guide to help you understand the facts about liposuction in order to make an informed decision about whether or not you might be a good candidate for the procedure.

In this book you will learn about:

- What liposuction is

- How it works

- The different forms of liposuction

- Who is a good candidate, who is not, and why

- What areas of the body can be treated

- Whether liposuction helps with cellulite and other skin irregularities

- How to find a qualified doctor

- Typical costs and whether insurance covers them

- What happens during a consultation

- How to prepare for the procedure
- What happens during liposuction surgery
- What happens after liposuction and how long it takes to recover
- Possible risks and complications
- Combining liposuction with other procedures, including fat injections
- When you need secondary procedures or "touch-ups"
- Psychological issues before and after surgery
- How to evaluate your results
- What to do if you are not happy with the results
- Whether or not the fat can come back to the same areas
- Liposuction procedures for men
- New and alternative liposuction procedures
- Other medical uses for liposuction
- How to take care of yourself before, during, and after surgery

We believe that a well-informed patient is the best patient. The more you know about liposuction before you make an appointment to see your doctor, the better your chances of achieving the results you want.

So if you have been carefully watching your weight and regularly exercising for years and are frustrated because that one area of fat simply will not come off, liposuction may be the solution you have been searching for. Because, as you will learn in this book, there are some fat deposits that will *never* come off with just diet and exercise.

With only a few hours in a doctor's office, using a modern liposuction technique with a very high safety record, you can lose the fat that has made you so unhappy for so many years. You can walk out with a new contour, one that will make your clothes fit better and your body look more pleasingly shaped.

By the time you finish this book, you will:

• Understand the advantages and risks of liposuction

• Know whether or not you may be a good candidate

• Have a realistic picture of the kinds of results you can expect to achieve

Today, modern liposuction techniques have an extremely high safety record and can produce amazing results. For examples, just have a look at the before-and-after photographs in this book. Hundreds of thousands of satisfied patients have made liposuction the single most popular cosmetic surgical procedure today.

So if you find yourself looking longingly at celebrities— or your friends—and asking, "Why can't I look that good?" the answer may well be "you can."

Come along on a journey with Dr. Ron Shelton, a highly experienced dermatologic surgeon who has performed hundreds of liposuction procedures. Through a simple question-and-answer format, Dr. Shelton will help you learn how liposuction, the amazing way to reshape your body, has helped so many women and men look better and whether or not you can become one of them.

1

• WHAT IS LIPOSUCTION?

WHEN liposuction first exploded in popularity several years ago, it was a frequent topic for television news and talk shows. However, as is often the case, many of these shows focused on the negative: stories about people who had unwanted complications during the early years when the technique was in its infancy.

In addition, the sight of a rather large tube sucking fat out of a hole in the body of an unconscious patient was hardly attractive. Even when the results were excellent and the patient looked considerably slimmer and happier, many viewers were simply turned off by the procedure they had seen.

Today, liposuction techniques have dramatically changed and improved. As you will see in this chapter, the procedure is now much safer and less complicated than in past years. So even if you think you know what's involved, it's quite possible that you have some wrong ideas.

Q: *What is liposuction?*

A: Liposuction is the removal of fat from the body using hollow, blunt-tipped tubes, called cannulas, that are connected to suction, whether by a syringe or an aspirator machine. Liposuction sculpts the body by removing unwanted fat—fat that does not respond to diet and exercise—from different areas. In fact, it's often called liposculpture for that reason. But it's important to know that liposuction is not a substitute for healthy diet and exercise, and it is not a method for losing weight.

Q: *Why is this procedure so popular?*

A: In a nutshell, there are certain locations on the body where diet and exercise cannot bring down that last bulge. In fact, too much exercise and too much dieting can be unhealthy, whether it's due to stress on the joints or interference with your quality of life as you spend hours in the gym, away from your family.

Using the liposuction procedure, significant amounts of fat can be removed through a small opening in the skin. This is usually done while patients are awake, and they can get up and go home shortly after the procedure is over. Recuperation is rather quick, and most people can resume their work and daily activities within a few days. But you also have to remember that liposuction is not a substitute for diet and exercise, and you have to continue with a healthy diet and exercise program afterward to maintain your results.

In short, liposuction is popular because it is a quick,

relatively painless way to remove stubborn pockets of fat that cannot be removed any other way.

Q: *What are the major areas of the body that can be treated with liposuction?*

A: The areas most frequently treated are the neck, arms, inner folds under the arms, upper back, belly, hips, thighs, buttocks, and the "love handles" and breasts (reduction) in men.

Q: *Is the procedure completely safe?*

A: Tumescent liposuction [see below] is extremely safe when you consider that it is the number-one cosmetic surgical procedure in the country. It does have some risks [see chapter thirteen]. There is not one surgical procedure that is without risks, but when it is performed on the proper candidate by an experienced physician using the proper technique, it is a very safe procedure. Not one fatality has been reported using pure tumescent liposuction.

Q: *Do liposuction patients feel pain during the procedure?*

A: Very rarely. Tumescent liposuction is done with local anesthetic. There may occasionally be some slight discomfort during the procedure, but there is no pain. In fact, a recent survey found that approximately three-quarters of liposuction patients who were questioned a week after surgery reported that they felt no discomfort at all during their procedure. Doctors vary in how they do the procedure and may provide no further medication, an anxiety-reducing pill, injections of painkillers, or sedatives.

However, not all doctors use the tumescent technique. Other doctors prefer to add general anesthesia or intravenous sedation, which means the patient may be completely unconscious during the procedure [see chapter eight].

Q: *What is tumescent liposuction?*

A: Tumescent liposuction uses local anesthesia and possible additions of anti-anxiety pills or intramuscular analgesics. It does not use general anesthesia or intravenous sedation. *Tumescence,* which is derived from a Latin word meaning "swelling" and is used medically to indicate a firm swelling, refers to the anesthetic that is used. This tumescent anesthetic causes swelling in the fatty tissue, minimizes blood loss, and allows patients to remain awake during the procedure so they can interact with their surgeons [see chapter eight].

Q: *Can you describe the best candidates for liposuction?*

A: Ideal candidates are those from their late 20s to their 50s who are not more than 10 or 20 pounds overweight and who do not have generalized obesity, meaning that the areas they want to reduce are clearly defined. These individuals should be healthy, involved in a regular exercise program, and have a diet that is well balanced [see chapter twenty]. They should not be taking any medication at the time of surgery that interferes with the metabolism of the local anesthetic [see chapter nine]. They should not have any disease that can increase the risk of local anesthetic toxicity or systemic infection, such as diabetes, liver disease, and certain heart conditions [see chapter four]. And women should not be pregnant or nursing when they have liposuction.

Q: *What kinds of expectations should ideal candidates have?*

A: It's very important to have realistic expectations when you undergo liposuction. You cannot expect to have a huge weight loss or go down several dress sizes. You have to realize that skin texture is not usually affected by liposuction, so cellulite, dimpling, and depressions will usually not improve. You should be aware that even though fat will be removed, you may only sense the difference after surgery by how your clothes fit, not by looking at your body, especially if only a small amount was removed.

Realistic patients have self-confidence and self-esteem and want to get rid of that last bulge because they realize they can't do it with diet and exercise. But they don't believe that once the unwanted fat is gone, their marital problems will disappear, their boyfriend will finally propose, or they will be able to get a better job or a raise at work. In other words, liposuction patients should not think of the procedure as a miracle-worker, but rather as a way to improve the contour of their bodies. They might not come out looking "perfect," but they will see a real improvement.

Q: *Can liposuction be performed on patients of all ages?*

A: Yes. In the early years, it was thought that the only good candidates were patients under 40, because of the youthfulness and elasticity of their skin. But in the years since, we have found that patients through their 70s can undergo liposuction with good results.

Q: *At what age do most people have liposuction?*

A: Very, very few teenagers have liposuction. A few people in their 20s have the procedure, but the numbers of people having liposuction peak for people in their 30s and 40s.

Q: *How long does the procedure usually take?*

A: The first visit or consultation takes about an hour [see chapter six]. The surgical liposuction procedure itself involves three parts: (1) preparation, (2) the procedure to remove the fat, and (3) application of the dressings afterward. The average patient is in the office for about five hours, but it can be more or less, depending on the procedure(s) being performed and the individual needs of each patient.

Q: *Where is liposuction usually performed?*

A: I do tumescent liposuction in my accredited office, as do many physicians. Liposuction is also done in ambulatory surgery centers and in hospital settings, depending on the type of procedure performed and the surgeon performing it.

Q: *How much time does a typical patient have to take off from work?*

A: It depends on what they do. If they have a very physical job—lots of manual labor, for example—they might need to take off for a week or more. People with desk jobs can often be back at work in two or three days. Again, it's an individual matter, with some patients taking longer to return and others going back sooner.

Q: *Approximately how long do the results last?*

A: The results of liposuction can last indefinitely. The procedure removes fat cells, not just the liquid fat. So if the patient maintains a good diet and exercise program after liposuction, there will probably be no return of the fat.

Q: *What happens if patients don't eat properly or fail to exercise regularly?*

A: Patients make a big mistake if they are careless and start eating more than they did before, or ignore their exercise regimen because they think they will have an "out" later on. They might think, *Oh, if I gain back any fat, I can just* *do more liposuction,* or, *You know what, I had liposuction, so I can cancel my gym membership and save that time and money to go shopping or go out with my friends.* Before you know it, they put the fat back on.

Q: *Does the fat return to the same areas where it was removed?*

A: It can, because even with the most extreme liposuction, not all the fat cells are removed. Some fat cells remain. So some of the fat they gain will go there, but proportionally. It is very rare that all the fat gained back goes into the area where it was surgically removed. Instead, it is distributed in a more general way.

Q: *Where does the new fat tend to go?*

A: There are some areas that are more resistant to diet and exercise. When you put weight on, then take it off, then put it on again, there are certain areas that tend to retain the fat. In women, it's often the belly and the outer thighs, while in men, it's the love handles (flanks). They tend to build up more and more each time there's an increase and decrease cycle.

Q: *Do many people gain weight after liposuction?*

A: Some do. One of the reasons is that after liposuction, you have reduced your weight and your fat stores. So if you go back to eating exactly what you ate before the surgery, it's quite possible that you will gain a little weight, because you no longer need the same number of calories as before. The best approach is to decrease your caloric intake and/or increase your exercise a little bit. If you do that, you should be able to maintain the correct weight and not put back on any weight.

Q: *Although liposuction is not intended for weight loss, does it help people lose weight?*

A: Yes, it does. The effect is not only physical, but psychological, as well. There have been reports of patients with realistic expectations who had problems trying to stick with their diet and exercise program before liposuction. But once they had one area done and saw the good results, they had a bigger incentive to maintain their program. They undergo the procedure and say, "Wow, look at me. There really is hope. After all these years, I finally reduced that bulge, it looks great, and I'm going to maintain it no matter what. I'm going to watch my diet, say no to that extra piece of cake, and go to the gym three times a week." And they do.

So we often find that people have greatly improved attitudes toward their bodies after liposuction, and that motivates them to keep the weight off and continue working to improve themselves.

Q: *What are the different forms of liposuction?*

A: The removal of body fat through liposuction can be done with a syringe or a machine. Both require at least a local anesthetic. Both types can provide good results, and physicians choose the approach they prefer.

Q: *What is the difference between syringe and machine-assisted liposuction?*

A: With syringe liposuction, you need nurses to constantly take the syringes from the surgeons and give them another syringe loaded with a cannula, which is a hollow cylinder; then the nurses have to empty the fat from the syringe and give the surgeons a fresh syringe. So the operating room could be a little messy as a result of all this activity.

It is also possible to lose the vacuum suction with a syringe if the opening gets too close to the opening of the skin. So surgeons sometimes have to spend extra time emptying the air out of the syringes and doing the steps over again.

With machine-assisted liposuction, you have a constant pressure, and usually that makes the procedure more efficient [see chapter eight for more details].

Q: *Can you describe the older forms of liposuction?*

A: In past years, liposuction was performed with what was called the "dry technique," using minimal anesthetic, or with the "wet technique," involving a dilute solution. But both of these procedures caused significant blood loss. As a result, in many cases there was a need for blood transfusions. And because of the need for general anesthesia, patients also had a higher rate of side effects and complications and often took longer to recover.

Q: *How is tumescent liposuction, the type that you perform, different?*

A: Tumescent liposuction is done without intravenous sedation or general anesthesia. It is performed with tumescent anesthesia, which makes the fat plump with rigidity and relatively easy to remove. Tumescent liposuction was designed by California dermatologic surgeon Dr. Jeffrey Klein [see chapter three] and is much safer than the older techniques.

Patients are given only local anesthesia, which means they are awake during the procedure and do not need blood transfusions. They bruise far less and are also able to turn over and assume different body positions with minimal assistance, making liposuction easier to perform.

Q: *What is superficial liposuction?*

A: Superficial liposuction refers to a procedure using smaller cannulas and is done by working higher up in the fatty compartment, near the skin level. The aim is to shape some of the muscular folds better, as well as get a more desirable overall effect. But if the surgeon goes too far, the procedure can cause complications such as scars or permanent changes in the skin texture. So it has to be done very carefully.

Q: *What is ultrasonic liposuction?*

A: Ultrasonic liposuction is liposuction using a special instrument to heat up and liquify the fat with ultrasonic energy so the fat can be more easily removed. The instrument used to do this can be used before or at the same time the fat removal is being performed. This technique is difficult to master.

Remember that surgeons are using a very hot instrument, so there is a risk of burns if it is not used correctly. Ultrasonic liposuction requires constant arm movements, and the surgeon cannot stop and rest in one position. The number of surgeons currently using this technique has decreased over the last several years.

Q: *What is powered liposuction?*

A: Powered liposuction often uses the tumescent technique. It involves a cannula that is moved not only by the surgeon's arms, but also has its own to-and-fro motion, which goes back and forth many times per second. This allows for greater removal of fat. Because the motion does not depend on the surgeon alone, it makes it easier on the surgeon's arms when working in certain areas such as the neck, where there is limited access, or around the belly button, where there is often a tendency for fat to remain.

Because powered liposuction allows the cannula to go back and forth so quickly, it is easier to get fat out of these more difficult areas of the body [see chapter eight for more details].

Q: *Is liposuction expensive?*

A: Remember that liposuction is a surgical procedure, so it usually runs in the thousands of dollars. Of course, fees vary according to such factors as where you live, who is doing your surgery, what procedures you undergo, how much fat has to be removed, and whether there is a lot of fibrous fat rather than soft fat. All these elements can have an effect on the price, which can vary from less than $2,000 to $6,000 or $8,000 and sometimes more.

Q: *Does insurance ever cover the cost of liposuction?*

A: No, not that I'm aware.

Q: *What is the general rate of patient satisfaction?*

A: A recent survey by the Accreditation Association for Ambulatory Health Care (AAAHC) found that among a group of patients who responded to a questionnaire six months after liposuction, 84 percent had a high level of satisfaction. In my personal experience, the rate of satisfaction is even higher.

Q: *About how many liposuction procedures are performed each year?*

A: No one knows exactly, because liposuction is an elective procedure and physicians are not required to report statistics to the government. One survey by the American Society of Plastic Surgeons found that in 2001, close to 200,000 liposuction procedures were performed. Today, that figure might well exceed 350,000 when you include figures from the American Academy of Cosmetic Surgery and the American Society for Dermatologic Surgery and allow for additional unreported procedures.

Q: *Who is the best doctor to perform liposuction, and is special training or certification required?*

A: The best doctor to do liposuction is a doctor who has experience with the procedure and whose patients and referring doctors are satisfied with that doctor's results. Liposuction can be performed by dermatologic surgeons and plastic surgeons. Both dermatology and plastic surgery teach the procedure to residents in training and it is part of the American Council of Graduate Medical Education (ACGME.) In other words, liposuction is a standard part of the training in both dermatology and plastic surgery. [See chapter five for more information.]

POINTS TO REMEMBER

- Liposuction is not a method for weight loss.

- Liposuction is designed to remove fat from parts of the body where it cannot be removed by diet and exercise alone.

- Liposuction is most frequently performed on the neck, arms, inner folds of the underarms, belly, hips, thighs, and buttocks. In men, the "love handles" and breasts are often reduced.

- Tumescent liposuction techniques have a very high record of safety.

- The procedure is not painful, except in rare circumstances, and at most, might cause slight discomfort while it is being performed.

- An ideal liposuction candidate is not very overweight, is healthy, eats a well-balanced diet, exercises, and has realistic expectations for the surgery.

- Liposuction can be performed on people of all ages, but is most often done on people between their 30s and 50s.

- The average time spent in the doctor's office for a procedure is five hours, but it can be more or less, depending on the procedure performed and other factors.

- Most people can return to work in a few days.

- Results can be permanent if patients follow the recommended program after having liposuction.

- There are different methods of performing liposuction. The tumescent is most commonly performed and does not require general anesthesia.

- Liposuction can vary in cost, from less than $2,000 to $8,000 or more, depending on where it is done and which procedure(s) are performed.

- Medical insurance does not cover liposuction.

- Dermatologic surgeons and plastic surgeons have training in and can both perform liposuction.

2
• WHAT LIPOSUCTION CAN AND CANNOT DO

IF you're like most people, you probably have some wrong ideas about liposuction. Yes, it can remove unwanted fat, but probably not as much as you imagine. Yes, it does recontour your body, but the results might not always be as dramatic as you think. No, you may not get the exact same results as your friend, even if she has a body and fat deposit exactly like yours. Yes, the results of liposuction can make you look much better and might even be permanent, but you have to work to keep it that way.

In short, you, like many other people, might not know precisely what liposuction can and cannot do. We will talk about some of your concerns in this chapter.

Q: *What are some of the realistic goals and expectations people should have before undergoing liposuction?*

A: The most realistic goal is to use liposuction to decrease a small volume of fat in an area that does not respond to persistent diet and exercise. If people are overweight from head to toe, then liposuction is not for them. But if they have a small projecting area of fat they are not able to bring down with diet and exercise, and it is in one of the common areas such as the neck, upper back, belly, hips, or thighs, then liposuction is quite possibly for them.

If someone has a problem with skin texture such as cellulite or dimpling or has unwanted depressions in the skin, liposuction will not make them better. You need to have a positive self-image, and there also has to be some real fat that needs to be removed. If people think they have fat that has to be removed and there really isn't any, they might have body image distortion, a psychological condition that makes people see themselves in a way that others do not see them—the condition that is linked to anorexia and bulimia in many young people.

But if you are healthy, exercise regularly, watch your diet, and just can't get your belly to go down and you want to have liposuction for that reason, you might well be a good candidate with realistic expectations.

Basically, liposuction can remove certain deposits of fat and recontour your body to give it a smoother outline. Some people will drop a dress size, but others might not look dramatically different. So although the procedure does not work miracles, it can have some wonderful results.

Q: *Can you get an idea of the results you're going to get by looking at your friends who have had the procedure?*

A: Only sometimes. Everyone is different. I've had different patients who have had similar body types in terms of where their fat deposits are located, but whose liposuction results were not the same. For instance, some people have more fibrous fat, some have wider bones, or some have more protruding muscles in the belly. All these things can affect the results.

So you can look at your friends or relatives and get some idea of what liposuction can do, but your own results might not turn out the same way. You can also look at photographs in the doctor's office to get an idea of what's possible, but you can't point to one and say, "Doctor, that's the one I want." In other words, you can get a general idea of what results you may get, but no one, including the surgeon, can know for certain until you actually have the procedure and start healing.

Q: *Why can't diet and exercise achieve the same results?*

A: Fat cells function differently in different parts of the body. The role of some is mainly to supply energy and metabolism. Other fat cells store energy for long-term starvation situations, and as a result, you will lose fat in your face before you lose fat around your love handles, lower belly, or outer thighs. Fat in these areas is more resistant, more stubborn. When you gain weight, it often goes there, and when you lose weight, it comes off of other areas. There is a real biochemical difference in the fat in different areas of the body.

In women, for example, it has been shown that the fat cells in the outer thighs are so resistant to diet and exercise that even a woman who is almost starving could put fat on in those areas in order to have reserves in case she should become pregnant or need to breast-feed.

Q: *What happens when people try to get this resistant type of fat off with exercise?*

A: They fail. Women will often say to me, "I have tried for five years to get rid of this fat. I've been working out for two hours every other day, or one hour every day, I have a good diet, and nothing I do will reduce my thighs." Or they tell me, "I've tried everything, and I just can't make my tummy go away."

But if they keep trying and they increase their exercise to four or five hours a day, they can run into physical problems with their joints. And of course, there are other important things most people want to do with their time than exercise. In the worst-case scenario, too much exercise in the pursuit of getting rid of stubborn fat deposits can become an obsession. It's an obsession that probably will not bring the results they want.

Q: *When fat deposits are removed with liposuction, are the results permanent?*

A: They can be if the patient remains very careful about diet and exercise. When the fat cells are removed, it does not mean you are taking the juice out of the cell and leaving the cell to reaccumulate fat. You are actually removing the fat cell itself, decreasing the population of fat cells in that spot. If you gain weight in the future, there is less of a chance that the fat is going to accumulate right there in the same spot where the fat cells were removed.

However, if someone becomes significantly overweight after liposuction, they can actually increase the number of fat cells again. They normally have to go up to 170 percent of their ideal body weight to do so. It's at that approximate weight that new fat cells begin to develop. So you can regain all the fat that liposuction has removed, but you have to gain quite a lot of weight to do it.

Q: *So in theory, you could get back to where you were before you had liposuction, even though it isn't likely?*

A: That's right. It would be more likely in people who are not good liposuction candidates, who do not have their weight under control with diet and exercise, who have an eating problem, and who are having the surgery just to get rid of excess weight. That's why it's so important to understand the purposes of liposuction and to be at or near your normal weight and stay there before and after the procedure. If you find yourself thinking, *I'm just going to take the easy way out, have liposuction and achieve my weight goal in a few hours, then go and celebrate by sitting home and eating donuts,* you will probably not benefit from the surgery.

Q: *Would you accept a patient like that?*

A: I would not, but not every doctor would turn such a person away.

Q: *Does liposuction have any effect on cellulite?*

A: For the most part, I tell my patients not to expect any improvement, but at times, there is some. There are also some very rare times when the cellulite looks worse after the procedure. Liposuction is not performed with the goal of making cellulite look better—that's not part of the procedure. If there's improvement, I'm happy. It's a gift. For patients who have significant cellulite, I prepare them by explaining that it might look better or possibly worse after surgery. For most people, cellulite does not change.

Q: *Is liposuction generally safe, or should people be concerned about possible complications?*

A: Tumescent liposuction is remarkably safe, but as with any surgical procedure, there are side effects that will occur. That doesn't mean it's not safe, however. For example, you have to be prepared for some form of mild tenderness, perhaps when you're moving around, sitting down, or doing some specific activity. That can last for a few days or more. There are also areas of the skin that might be numb for a while, and some people can develop skin that is extremely sensitive or itchy. Overall, though, the rate of serious complications or permanent problems is exceedingly low. [See chapter thirteen for more information.]

Q: *We know that liposuction is not a weight loss treatment, but how much weight do most people actually lose after the procedure?*

A: Fat is not a dense structure in the body, so when we remove fat through liposuction, we are usually not removing much weight. If you were to lose the equivalent volume in muscle mass, you would notice a significant weight change. But a woman who goes down one or two waist sizes via liposuction might not lose more than a pound or two. Some people might lose a bit more, perhaps up to five pounds, but most liposuction patients are not going to notice a very big change on the scale.

Q: *Do people ever regret having liposuction?*

A: On rare occasions, they have. Among the varied surgeons performing liposuction, there is a very small percentage of patients who, over the years, have had complications from the surgery. Some of these cases resulted from procedures that were too aggressive and removed too much fat, which can cause ulcerations in the skin, significant depressions, or long-standing discoloration, but such results are very unusual [see chapter thirteen].

Others might sometimes get uneven results, where one side has a little more fat removed than the other and they end up looking asymmetric. Or perhaps they were asymmetric before the procedure and the difference is just more noticeable afterward. Surgeons naturally try to correct any asymmetry during the procedure by removing less fat from the area that has less to begin with.

When people get these and the other kinds of complications we will discuss later, they might naturally regret having the surgery. But in my experience, this kind of situation is extremely rare. Most patients are very happy with their results and wonder why they waited so long to have liposuction.

Q: *Can liposuction change a person's life?*

A: Yes, of course it can, usually in small ways, but occasionally in significant ways. For a few people, the extra self-confidence they feel can have a kind of ripple effect, leading them to many other positive changes in their lives. But of course, no one should decide to have liposuction in order to change their life!

After liposuction, most patients feel happier and more self-confident. They're pleased that they finally decided to go ahead and have the procedure, and they're happy that they finally built up the courage to do it. For these people, their typical reaction during the treatment is, "This isn't bad at all. I can't believe I waited so long."

Q: *What were the factors that made them put it off for so long?*

A: There are a number of things. One is all the "horror stories" that were circulating several years ago when liposuction was first introduced. Another is not knowing what the procedure will feel like—they have anxiety about pain or a lengthy recovery period. That's why it is so important for people to be well informed. Then they will know that a lot of what the media have told them about liposuction is not accurate—especially today—and they will feel more confident knowing the facts and exactly what to expect.

POINTS TO REMEMBER

- Liposuction will decrease the volume of fat, but usually not by a large amount.

- Liposuction is not intended for those who are very overweight or obese.

- If you have a fat deposit that does not respond to diet and exercise and you are healthy, you might be a good candidate for liposuction.

- Everyone is different, and it is not possible to precisely predict what results you will get.

- In women, the major areas treated are the lower belly, outer thighs, hips, neck, buttocks, upper back, inner thighs, back of the thighs, and front of the thighs.

- In men, the major areas treated are the love handles and the breasts (reduction).

- Fat cells in certain body areas retain their fat, even when there is a weight loss.

- Fat removal with liposuction can be permanent if the individual maintains proper weight through diet and exercise. Otherwise, some of the fat might return, but a great deal of weight has to be gained before it returns to the way it was before the procedure.

- Liposuction does not usually have any effect on cellulite, but on some occasions, it can make it a little better or a little worse.

- Liposuction is a remarkably safe procedure, although like any surgical procedure, it does have some possible side effects.

- With most procedures, a pound or two of weight may be lost. Patients rarely lose more than five pounds.

- Most people are very glad that they had liposuction and wish they had done it sooner. A very small number who have complications may have regrets.

- Liposuction can have a positive effect on one's life, increasing self-esteem and providing motivation for continued self-improvement.

- Stories in the media have occasionally frightened people regarding liposuction, creating unwarranted anxieties. Patients who are well informed about the procedure understand that it is not dangerous, painful, or otherwise anxiety-provoking.

3

• THE HISTORY OF LIPOSUCTION

Q: *How long have physicians been performing liposuction?*

A: In the mid-1970s, Drs. Arpad and Giorgio Fischer, Italian father and son cosmetic surgeons, first developed the liposuction technique, although their procedure was very different from the tumescent liposuction we use today. They invented a blunt, hollow tube which they attached to suction. Some of these tubes also had blades to cut into the fat. Prior to their invention, unwanted fat was removed by cutting into it with a scalpel or curette, which often resulted in excessive bleeding, uneven results, and other complications.

Q: *How did liposuction techniques develop?*

A: In the late 1970s, liposuction became very popular throughout Europe. A French physician, Dr. Gerald Illouz, made some changes in the Fischers' method and eventually developed the "wet technique," using an injected solution before suctioning out the fat. Another French physician, Dr. Pierre Fournier, also refined the Fischers' techniques, although he initially preferred a "dry technique," with no fluids injected before fat suctioning. Later on, Fournier adopted the wet technique.

Q: *When was liposuction introduced into this country?*

A: During the 1970s, American physicians were aware of the growing popularity of liposuction, and many of them observed the procedure and its results in Europe. Then, in the mid-1980s, American physicians went to Europe to train with Drs. Illouz and Fournier.

Q: *When was the tumescent technique developed?*

A: Dr. Jeffrey Klein, a California dermatologic surgeon, developed the tumescent technique in 1985 using local anesthetic for the liposuction procedure. The low concentration of the anesthetic he injected permitted the numbing of a much larger area than had been previously possible with local anesthetic. By avoiding the risks of general anesthesia, the tumescent technique achieved a much higher rate of safety. It also meant that liposuction could be performed outside of a hospital setting, which is much more convenient for both the patient and the doctor.

Q: *When did liposuction become so popular?*

A: In the early years, when liposuction was performed only in hospitals using general anesthesia, the side effects and complications kept many people from having it. So the current popularity of liposuction really started after Dr. Klein's introduction of the tumescent technique. Once people saw that they could spend just a few hours in a doctor's office, remain awake, have a painless and very safe procedure, and return home for a few days' recuperation, they were much more willing to try it. And of course today we also have power-assisted liposuction, which has been available since 2000. When we look at how many people are now undergoing this procedure, I think the numbers speak for themselves.

4

• ARE YOU A GOOD CANDIDATE?

AS wonderful as liposuction sounds, it is not for everyone. Some people are excellent candidates and will benefit from the procedure, others might not get good results, and still other people, for various reasons, should never have liposuction.

Are you a good candidate? This chapter will help you find out. We will discuss what factors might make liposuction right for you and what factors might rule it out. And if you don't qualify now but think you might like to try it in the future, you will learn what you can do to improve your status. You will also find out why it is so important for prospective liposuction patients to be as well informed about the procedure as possible, so keep reading!

Q: *What are some of the characteristics that make some-one a good candidate for liposuction?*

A: Prospective patients can be of almost any age, from their 20s to their 80s, but they must be in good health. The ideal patient is a person who has been trying for some time to lose excess weight with diet and exercise, but has not been able to remove the last inch from a specific area. The most common of those difficult areas are the chin and neck, upper back, belly, hips, love handles, buttocks, and thighs.

Q: *How can you tell if the fat that is bothering you in those areas will come off with liposuction?*

A: One thing you can look for is whether these places are discrete areas, meaning areas that have a border that a physician can easily determine, so there is something obvi-ous to work on. In other words, these areas should not blend into one another in a pattern of overall excess fat.

If people don't like their overall contour and feel they are simply too big all over and they haven't been working out regularly or eating a healthy diet, liposuction would not be a good choice to improve things.

Q: *So you really need to have a definite area of excess fat that can be easily seen?*

A: Yes, that's right. Otherwise, when you do liposuction, you can't get a good transition to the adjacent areas. In other words, if a person is generally overweight, how can the physician know where to stop?

Q: *What is an ideal weight for a good liposuction candidate?*

A: The ideal candidate should be no more than 10 to 20 pounds overweight at most and preferably less. Of course, this person doesn't need to be overweight at all and is often someone who has been exercising for a long time to try to get rid of that last little bulge that refuses to go away.

Each person's ideal weight depends on their height and build, so you have to look at a chart to get the correct weight range for each person. For liposuction, it's preferable that someone is not more than 20 pounds over their ideal weight.

Q: *Does that mean someone who is more than 20 pounds overweight can't have liposuction?*

A: No. Overweight people can have liposuction in many areas. One of the more common areas I have operated on in overweight people is the neck. Even if people diet and exercise, they are not going to lose much in the neck area, because the chances are that it's an inherited tendency. They have probably noticed a double chin since they were in their teens or early 20s, similar to someone else in their family.

Q: *Is it true that younger patients are better candidates? Aren't elasticity of the skin and faster healing important factors for recovering from surgery?*

A: There is no doubt that elasticity is better at a younger age than at an older age especially if someone has, with time, developed irregular indentations in the skin and a lack of recoil so the skin isn't taut. Liposuction on those people can sometimes accentuate their skin irregularities. They will get volume reduction and be happier with how their clothes fit, but they might not look dramatically better when they put on a bathing suit. So in that sense, younger patients can have better results.

But you also have to remember that people age differently and their chronological age doesn't always tell you how much they have aged physically. So the old rule of no liposuction for people over 40 has long been thrown out. Many people who are in their 50s still have a good deal of skin elasticity.

It also depends on which areas are being done. The thighs or belly that has lost a lot of weight might have a very bad skin tone; stretch marks; indentations; cellulite; or loose, flabby skin. Liposuction can really reduce the girth of hanging fat, but the skin might not look as attractive as those who have more youthful skin.

Q: *What are some of the health conditions that would rule out liposuction or make it questionable?*

A: Certainly any chronic disease that affects the immune system could rule you out. Or it might be because you're on a medication for rheumatoid arthritis such as Prednisone. If you have a chronic immune deficiency disorder, diabetes, or chronic skin infections, you would be more at risk for developing an infection if you had liposuction. If you have heart problems such as angina or have had a heart attack, there is a risk that the local anesthetic, which has adrenaline in it, might bring on a further heart problem. Artificial heart valves could also be a problem, and many people who have them are on medication such as the blood thinner Coumadin. If you have had a stroke, that would not make you a good liposuction candidate; stroke patients are also very often on blood thinning medications and doctors would not want to take them off their medication just so they could have an elective procedure.

There can also be problems with patients who have kidney failure or liver disease. The liver is particularly important because of the way it metabolizes the anesthetic; with liver disease, the anesthetic hangs around longer, which can increase to a toxic level.

Because of these and other potential complications, it is very important that liposuction patients fully inform their doctors about any and all health conditions, past and present, and any medications they may be taking or have taken recently.

Q: *Can women who are pregnant or breast-feeding have liposuction?*

A: No, any woman who is pregnant or breast-feeding should not have liposuction.

Q: *What are some of the medications, herbs, and vitamins that people should avoid prior to liposuction?*

A: There is a very long list of prescription and over-the-counter medications, vitamins, and herbs that can interfere with liposuction. I give my patients this list, and if they are taking any of the substances, they must inform me. They include nonsteroidal anti-inflammatory medications such as Motrin, Advil, Ibuprofen, Clinoril, Vioxx, Celebrex, Voltaren, Anaproxin, and Naprosyn. Also aspirin and aspirin-containing medication can interfere with liposuction.

As for vitamins and herbs, those to avoid include vitamin E, ginseng, garlic tablets, ginkgo, and ginger. All these and certain others increase the tendency to bleed during a procedure and could cause unwanted complications. It's extremely important to inform your surgeon if you are taking any of them. That includes street drugs as well, such as cocaine, because cocaine stimulates the heart, and if it is in the system while the patient is given adrenaline, there can be serious consequences.

Q: *Do people taking the items on this list have to stop taking them?*

A: That depends. If they are medications that are necessary for their health and well-being, it might not be a good idea to stop taking them. That's something that you and your doctor have to work out on an individual basis. For others, it is often possible to stop taking them for a specific period of time before and after liposuction. For example, I ask my patients to stop taking aspirin and its derivatives, vitamin E, and certain herbs for as much as two weeks before surgery.

Q: *What are some psychological factors that would make someone a good candidate for liposuction?*

A: A good psychological profile would be someone who is largely happy with themselves and their lives, who is content with the people in their lives, and who is contemplating liposuction in order to improve a localized situation that they do not consider the focus of any personal problems.

Q: *What if someone* does *consider that pocket of fat to be a major problem?*

A: Once they consider a spot to be the focus of their problems, something else is going on. If the situation is extreme enough, that is, people are very overweight and feel that their lover or spouse is not paying enough attention to them, or that they can't find a boyfriend or girlfriend who finds them attractive, liposuction is not going to be the answer.

Or if they aren't very overweight but believe that once they have that last little bulge removed with liposuction their boyfriend or girlfriend will stay with them or their spouse won't leave them, in all likelihood, something else is going on. They are transferring their personal problems to a bit of extra fat.

Q: *Do people sometimes experience depression following surgery?*

A: Yes, a mild form of depression often occurs with cosmetic procedures. And patients have to be psychologically prepared for it. A couple days after surgery, people might say, "Why did I do this? Look at me. I'm bruised, I'm swollen, and I can't go to the beach for a few weeks. Why did I do this to myself?" It's a normal reaction, especially if there is a little soreness. In almost every case, it goes away pretty quickly. Good candidates understand this and can handle it well.

Q: *What happens if patients are already suffering from depression prior to surgery?*

A: That can be a big problem, especially if they think that liposuction is the answer to all their difficulties. Then, even if they are told what to expect following surgery and they understand that there might be some soreness and bruising, they can still get very depressed and it can last for a while.

Q: *Why is it so important for patients to be informed about liposuction in advance?*

A: People need to know about the procedure, and they have to be aware of and fully informed about the indications, the reasons why they might benefit from liposuction, the actual treatment, and what it's going to be like, including the convalescent period. This information helps them decide whether liposuction is right for them and if they are likely to achieve their goals. Could a better diet and more exercise achieve the same result? What will happen if they don't have the procedure? What are they going to look like if they do have it?

People need to know, because if they don't, they can experience anxiety about what is going to happen, which can be far worse than the actual experience itself. So I become concerned if someone tells me, "Don't bore me with the details. I know you're a good doctor, my friends recommended you, and I don't need to hear any medical details. Just book me, do the procedure, and get it over with. I'm sure I'll be fine."

Q: *What is your approach to keeping your patients well informed?*

A: I don't want my patients to bury their heads in the sand. I want them to be fully informed about liposuction and understand everything that will happen, because my patients are partners in a team approach. Doctors can't do everything by themselves. There has to be cooperation among everyone involved—the doctor, nurses, assistants, office staff, and, of course, the patient.

Q: *What kind of attitude does the ideal patient have toward the surgery?*

A: An ideal candidate has realistic expectations and knows that any form of surgery has some risks and possible complications. They understand the limitations of liposuction and realize that liposuction can help remove their stubborn areas of fat but will probably not improve their cellulite, irregular skin, dimpling, and depressions; nor will they lose a great deal of weight.

The best liposuction patients are those who take good care of themselves, have consistently maintained a good diet and exercise program, and will continue to follow it after the procedure. In addition, these patients are undergoing liposuction to please themselves, not someone else. They are doing it for self-improvement, not to replace the loss of a loved one or a job or anything else. They have good self-esteem and want to deal with something that can be improved using a very safe surgical procedure.

Q: *Please describe the realistic expectations of good candidates.*

A: Good liposuction candidates are not looking for weight loss on the scale, but are rather looking to feel and look better in clothing (and perhaps a bathing suit) by removing a deposit of fat that will not go away with diet and exercise. Afterward, they hope to look the way they imagine themselves, but they also understand that results can not be predicted precisely.

Q: *What questions can candidates ask themselves to try to figure out if liposuction is right for them?*

A: They can ask themselves *Am I really reducing my caloric intake? Have I given it my best without starving myself? Am*

*I just skipping meals and then bingeing? Am I replacing a
healthy meal with ice cream? Am I having extra portions of
pasta with dinner? Am I exercising enough?*

I have found that many people, whether they realize it
or not, are not completely honest about their lifestyles.
They might say, "I get plenty of exercise," but when you
question them closely, it turns out that they walk on the golf
course instead of taking a cart, or they walk to the train sta-
tion. That's good, but it's not sustained exercise where the
heart rate is elevated enough. So although it's better than
no exercise at all, it is not the best exercise. It probably will
not reduce their fat.

Then, if they are doing all the things they should be
doing and have reduced their fat to a point where they hon-
estly believe they can't reduce it any further, they can ask
themselves, *Is there anything else I can do to get rid of this
last bit of fat?* If the answer is really *No, not on my own,*
then they can conclude that they are not using liposuction
as a substitute for diet and exercise. These people might be
very good candidates.

Q: *Is there a way to tell whether or not that last bit of fat can
or cannot be lost any other way?*

A: First of all, you really need to work at diet and exercise
for at least 6 to 12 months. If you've only been working at it
for two or three months, you're not going to lose that much
weight. We know that the majority of weight loss at the
beginning of a diet is fluid loss, and that is not what we're
talking about.

So you need to stick with it. You absolutely should not

go on a crash diet before liposuction, because it can deplete your body of essential nutrients. Proper weight loss takes time. To some extent, a medical examination can reveal what is localized fat versus what is generalized fat. If a person is determined to have generalized obesity, he or she is not a good liposuction candidate. If he or she has localized obesity, then it's very possible he or she is a good candidate.

POINTS TO REMEMBER

- Liposuction is most commonly performed on people from their 30s through their 50s, but younger and older people can also be good candidates.

- Patients should be in good health. Certain medical conditions mean that the patient should not have liposuction, due to the risks.

- Ideal patients should have followed a good diet and exercise program for at least six months to a year and have just one or two small bulges remaining that they cannot reduce.

- The most common areas where stubborn fat exists are the chin, neck, upper back, belly, hips, love handles, buttocks, and thighs.

- Fat to be removed by liposuction should be in a clearly defined area, not a part of overall obesity or overweight.

- The ideal patient is not more than 10 to 20 pounds overweight.

- Some medications rule out liposuction. Others, including

over-the-counter drugs, vitamins, and herbs, must be stopped for a specific time period before and after liposuction.

- Pregnant and breast-feeding women should not have liposuction.

- The ideal patient has no deep psychological disorders and has a positive and realistic attitude toward the procedure, knowing it will not solve personal problems.

- A short period of minor psychological depression is not uncommon following surgery.

- The ideal patient is very well informed about liposuction prior to undergoing the procedure and is an active part of the health-care team.

- Realistic expectations include not expecting a great weight loss from liposuction and understanding that precise results can not be known until after the surgery.

5

• HOW DO YOU FIND A GOOD DOCTOR?

AT this point, you may have already decided that you are a good candidate for liposuction. But how do you find the right doctor? Liposuction is a special procedure that is performed only by certain doctors. Even so, there are many qualified doctors, especially if you live in or near a major urban area. How do you find the one who is right for you— a physician who is experienced and can help you get the results you want? In this chapter, you will learn how to carry out your search and which tools can help you along the way.

Q: *Which medical professionals are qualified to perform liposuction?*

A: Both dermatologic surgeons and plastic surgeons are qualified to perform liposuction, and both receive training during their medical residencies. But just because physicians have been exposed to some training, does not necessarily mean they are fully qualified to perform it well.

A physician needs actual hands-on liposuction experience to attain a good level of skill. That experience should be supplemented with continuing medical education such as attending conferences, watching videotapes, participating in live surgery workshops sponsored by medical societies, and, most important, observing experienced surgeons first-hand. If possible, they should even have these experienced surgeons at their side for advice when they perform their first few procedures.

So although other types of physicians may perform liposuction, dermatologists and plastic surgeons are the two most common and widely accepted specialists in the field.

Q: *Is there any special medical certification required for liposuction?*

A: No, not at this time.

Q: *What are the best ways for potential patients to find a good doctor?*

A: Without a doubt, the best way is to get a referral from a friend or relative who has had liposuction and is happy with the surgeon and the results. Many times, however, patients are not very willing to tell people they have had the surgery. But if someone you know does tell you or someone else, it's a good idea to contact that person and ask some questions.

Q: *What should you ask?*

A: Did you like the doctor? Did you like the staff? What was the procedure like? Were your needs met? Were your concerns addressed? Were your questions answered? Did you get a response when you called after hours? If you needed a follow-up appointment, was it scheduled in a timely fashion? If you had any special concerns following surgery, were you able to contact the doctor and have your concerns addressed and resolved quickly?

Q: *What do the answers to these questions tell us about the doctor and the office?*

A: Although it is very important to have a technically excellent physician, it is also important to have a physician who is communicative and responsive to your concerns, as well as an office staff that works closely with the doctor and makes sure contact is made when you need help.

Q: *So a prospective patient is looking not only at the individual physician, but also at the whole office staff and how it operates?*

A: Correct. A doctor might be very good at surgery, but if you leave an important message and it never gets through to the doctor, that doesn't help you. Many people don't think about these things in advance, but they are very important aspects of medical care, and you want to ask your friends about them as part of their referral.

Q: *What other sources can help you find a good doctor?*

A: You can ask your primary care physician for a referral. Or you can contact any of the organizations listed in the Resources section at the end of this book and request referrals for qualified doctors in your area. But these organizations do not grade or select the best doctors to perform any specific procedure. The names you get from these organizations are doctors who have taken a special interest in doing cosmetic procedures and have taken the extra effort to become a member of a specialty society. They might be doing some liposuction, but you don't know how much experience they have or how good they are at the procedure.

Another way is to use the Internet and go through the websites of some physicians who perform liposuction. Sometimes you can get an idea of their practice from the information you find there.

Q: *If friends refer you to their liposuction surgeons and tell you they were very happy with the results, is that good enough?*

A: It's a good start, but you might want to do a little more research. For instance, you can check with your primary care physician and ask if they know the doctors or have heard anything positive or negative. You can call the doctors' offices and find out if they are board certified [meaning they have fully completed their specialty training and have taken and passed a test administered by peers], which can be a plus. You can ask how many years they have been in practice, how long they have done the procedure, how many procedures they have performed, and what kind of training they have—all these are important questions.

Not every doctor who performs liposuction well is board certified, but if they are board certified in dermatologic surgery or plastic surgery, it is an indication they have completed some formal graduate training, have experience in their specialty, and are accepted by their peers.

Q: *Should prospective patients specifically seek out a doctor who is board certified?*

A: Not necessarily. There are surgeons who perform wonderful surgery before they become board certified. But if they have certification, that means they have a certain amount of experience in their specialty, and more experience almost always makes for a better physician. But there are also surgeons who are board certified and who might not be the best choices for you. Board certification is only one consideration and should not be the only factor in your decision.

Q: *Is it ever possible to talk with a doctor on the phone before making an appointment to come in?*

A: To the best of my knowledge, only a very small number of doctors will talk to prospective patients they have never met. Some physicians give consultations on the web, but they charge for them. In both cases, I think there is a danger of giving advice to people you have never seen or examined, so most physicians don't want to do that. You really need to meet in person and establish a physician-patient relationship.

For example, if I talk to you on the phone, I have no proper documentation, because there is no patient chart. I can't examine you and give you an informed opinion about what treatment you might or might not need. Then, if I see you a few months later, I have no way of remembering everything that was discussed.

Q: *How can a prospective patient make judgments about a doctor?*

A: The most important way to do that is to make an appointment for a consultation and meet your surgeon in person. A surgeon may be technically wonderful, but if you can't develop a bond or rapport or feel comfortable in the presence of that surgeon, that could be a warning sign. Patients need more from a doctor than just technical expertise. They need someone who is responsive to their needs, especially at the times when it is most important. Calling a physician and talking on the phone cannot provide you with knowledge about whether or not a rapport is there. I don't think you have anything to gain by speaking to a doctor on the phone about liposuction. You need to go into the office and meet.

Q: *What kind of printed information will a doctor's office send you?*

A: You have to ask about what they have available. Some offices don't have any printed material or only limited brochures and nothing on liposuction. They may do the procedure and do it well, but they may not be as concerned with communication skills as other offices.

In our office, we have spent a lot of time over the years constantly updating and modifying our patient handouts, and we always take our patients' comments into consideration. We love to send this information out to patients who express an interest. We also refer them to our website, and we have a patient coordinator who will speak with them on the phone. So a phone call to a prospective doctor's office can get very good results, depending on what is available in that office.

Q: *What are some other ways to get information from the office?*

A: General questions about liposuction can often be answered by a member of the office staff, such as a nurse or patient coordinator, and printed information can be mailed or faxed to you or may be available on the doctor's website.

Q: *When it comes to physicians who administer Botox, very often many of the office staff have tried it. Is the same true of liposuction?*

A: No. Botox is a much less invasive procedure, and not as many people have had liposuction, which is surgery. But if you want to talk to someone who has undergone the procedure, you should ask at the office. There are people in our office who have had it and are willing to answer patient questions. It's a good way to get information, so remember to ask about it when you come in to the doctor's office.

Q: *How many doctor candidates should a patient talk to before deciding on one?*

A: I don't think you need to have a second opinion if you've talked to one physician and you're happy with what you've heard—especially if you are already well informed about liposuction. You can come into the office prepared with good questions for the doctor, know exactly what you are looking for, then decide if you have found it.

There are some people who may like what they hear with the first physician they meet, but somehow, something doesn't feel quite right or they don't feel entirely comfortable. In a case like that, it makes sense to meet with another physician.

Q: *What are some of the things that might make someone feel that not everything is quite right?*

A: There could be many reasons. Maybe they don't like the price; maybe they think the postoperative instructions are too restrictive; maybe they like the doctor but they didn't get the right feeling from another staff member. There could be any number of reasons that would make someone think twice. And there's nothing wrong with that. You should feel very satisfied before you make a commitment to have surgery.

So the bottom line is this: If you find someone who comes well recommended and you have very good rapport with that doctor, you don't really need a second opinion. You will know in your heart when you feel comfortable and ready to proceed.

Q: *How much experience with liposuction should a doctor have?*

A: I think the surgeon should have done at least fifty procedures. In my experience, after the first twenty-five procedures, you are already getting pretty good at it. Of course, there are surgeons who have done hundreds of liposuction procedures and some who have done thousands. But there is a learning curve, and most people would not want to be one of a doctor's first ten patients, because you might not get the best results.

Q: *Do doctors ever give patients a free consultation?*

A: Some doctors do, but not many. In some offices, they charge a consultation fee and if the patient decides to have the procedure, it is deducted from the cost of the procedure. You have to ask each office about their individual policy.

Q: *Because there are different forms of liposuction, does the type the doctor performs have any influence on the patient's decision?*

A: Yes, it does influence their decision.

Q: *So it's important to ask doctors what type of liposuction they perform?*

A: That's right. There are still doctors who put their patients to sleep and do not do tumescent liposuction. There are a number of reasons why some patients might prefer this, including the fact that some patients know themselves and do not want to be awake during the procedure. So finding out what liposuction method a surgeon uses is an important part of making an informed decision. [See chapter eight for a discussion of the different forms of liposuction.]

Q: *Is it a good idea for people to use a cosmetic/plastic surgery consulting firm to find a good doctor?*

A: A good consulting firm can be very helpful. Cosmetic consultants are usually not physicians, but they may have

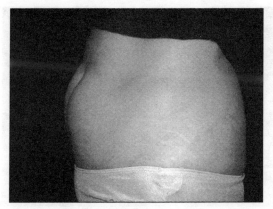

Before abdominal liposuction

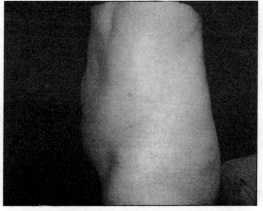

Immediately after abdominal liposuction

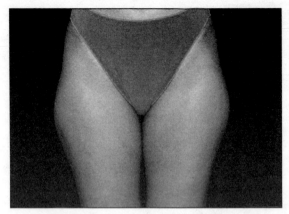

Before outer thigh and buttock liposuction

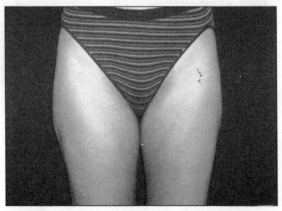

17 weeks after outer thigh and buttock liposuction

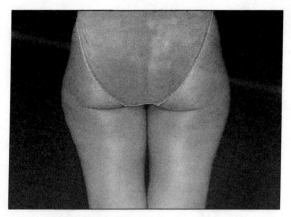

Before outer thigh and buttock liposuction

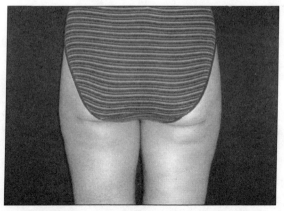

17 weeks after outer thigh and buttock liposuction

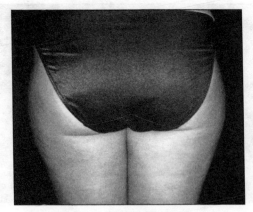

Before outer thigh liposuction

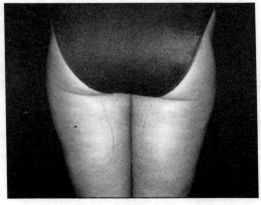

1 month after outer thigh liposuction

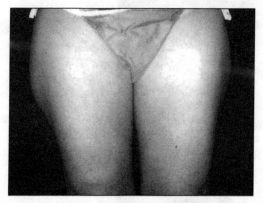

Before outer thigh liposuction

(Please note asymmetrically larger right saddlebag)

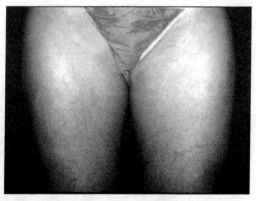

2 weeks after outer thigh liposuction

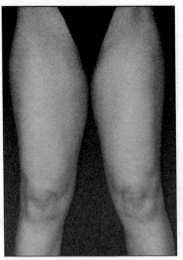

Before liposuction
of inner thigh
and inner knee

7 months after
liposuction
of inner thigh
and inner knee

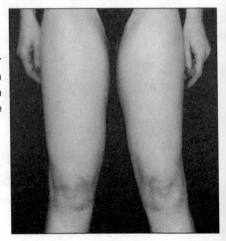

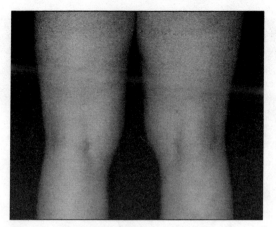

Before liposuction of inner knee

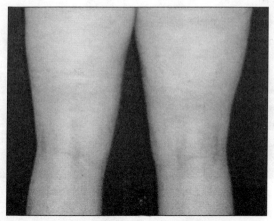

11 weeks after liposuction of inner knee

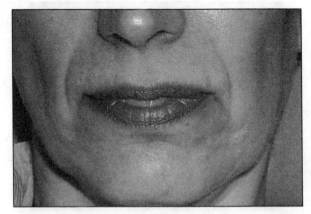

Before fat augmentation of mid-cheeks and smile folds

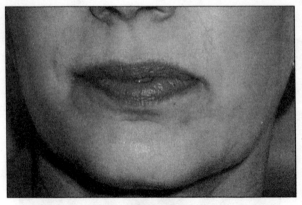

One week after fat augmentation of mid-cheeks
and smile folds

worked in a surgeon's office and/or had procedures done themselves and are quite familiar with the intricacies of cosmetic surgery and postoperative convalescence. They also know a great deal about cosmetic surgery practices and can work with you to find the surgeon who best suits your needs. Of course, consultants charge a fee for their services. They listen to your concerns, interests, and goals and then try to match you with a doctor who they think would be right for you. They usually provide you with more than one name, and you take it from there.

POINTS TO REMEMBER

- Dermatologic surgeons and plastic surgeons are both qualified to perform liposuction.

- A referral from a physician or a friend who has had liposuction and liked his or her doctor is the best way to find a good surgeon.

- You should ask your friend for detailed information about the doctor, the office, and the procedure.

- Doctors' communication skills can be just as important as their technical skills.

- You can also get referrals from your primary care physician, professional organizations, and the Internet.

- Board certification is a plus, but is not always a necessity.

- You can request printed information from the doctor's office and sometimes talk to a nurse or patient coordinator regarding your questions.

- It is essential to have personal rapport with your doctor and feel comfortable in his or her presence.

- If you are happy with the first doctor you meet, it is not essential for you to seek out other candidates.

- It is best to find a doctor who has performed at least 50 liposuction procedures.

- Ask the doctor what form of liposuction he or she performs, because it can influence your decision.

- Cosmetic/plastic surgery consulting firms can be very helpful in matching you with a surgeon.

6

• YOUR FIRST VISIT TO THE DOCTOR

BY now, you know what liposuction is, what it can do, and what makes a good candidate. You've decided that you are seriously interested in liposuction and have found at least one, and perhaps more, potential doctors. Your next step is to make an appointment for a consultation so the doctor can examine you, talk with you about your concerns, find out why you want liposuction, and let you know what can be done. In this chapter, you will learn what happens at your consultation or first visit, what you can do in advance to make this first meeting more productive, what questions you should ask the doctor, and what questions the doctor might ask you.

Q: *Is your first visit to the doctor always a consultation?*

A: Yes, it is.

Q: *What should a patient bring along for this first visit, or consultation?*

A: It's a good idea to bring a written list of your questions, so you won't forget anything. I like to explain the procedure to patients and when I'm finished, have them ask me questions. If there are certain things they bring up that I haven't discussed, it helps me to think about them and possibly discuss them with future patients.

That's all you really need to bring. You don't have to bring pictures of yourself, but you can do that if you have a specific reason. For example, if there is some fat on your neck that you want trimmed down and you have a photograph of how it used to look, that can be helpful for the doctor. We might not be able to get it back to exactly the way it was before, but photos give us a clear idea of what the patients want. Then we can show the patients what we think we can do, so they will have realistic expectations.

Q: *Is it a good idea to ask the office to send forms to your home in advance so you can arrive with them already filled out?*

A: Some offices may do that. It depends on how many days in advance you make your appointment. You can also have them faxed or e-mailed to you, but some patients prefer to fill them out when they come in to the office. Some patients fill out the forms at home and forget to bring them in. But if the office is willing to send them and you want to save a little time, you can ask about it. Of course, you can't fill out everything in advance. In my office, there is a substantial number of forms to fill out, including your medical history, much of which is taken down verbally.

Q: *What other forms have to be filled out?*

A: There is a demographic form with the patient's address and phone number; there's also a patient's medical history form listing any medications they're taking, any allergies to medication, and any vitamins or herbs they take. Then there are forms that the nurse and doctor fill out when they interview and examine the patient. These include notes on the physical examination, plans about what will be done during the liposuction surgery, a quote sheet for the fees, and a consent form they can read so they will be fully informed of any possible side effects or complications that could occur.

Q: *Do patients have to sign the consent form at the consultation?*

A: No. It is signed prior to the actual procedure as a consent for the surgery. Patients are also informed that they have to have someone to go home with, that they cannot go home and stay there alone following liposuction surgery. [See chapters nine and twelve.]

Q: *After the patients fill out the forms, what happens next?*

A: In my office, they meet with the nurse first. The nurse takes some of their history and finds out why they are there. If they want liposuction, the nurse will ask where on the body they want it and what they hope to achieve. They are also asked about their normal weight, their maximum weight, their ideal weight, what kind of diet they eat, what exercise program they follow, if they are pregnant or nursing, and so on.

We have an extensive checklist that helps us make sure we take a very complete history for every patient. We have the same routine for the physical examination, because no matter how many patients you see and how experienced you are, you can't afford to forget anything.

Q: *Do patients have to bring past medical records with them?*

A: No, that's not necessary. If they are needed, they can be acquired later on.

Q: *What kinds of medical conditions would you be concerned about?*

A: We have to watch for easy bruising, hemophilia factor 8 deficiency, or anything that would make people bleed easily or cause them to have trouble with normal clotting. We need to find out if people have any of the above or a history of blood clots, deep vein thrombosis, phlebitis, liver disease, diabetes, immunosuppression, artificial joints, and artificial heart valves. Also, we need to know if people have significant cardiovascular disease, peripheral vascular disease, any form of bad arterial circulation, thyroid disease, or adrenal tumors. We also look at surgical scars to see how they have healed. If we feel we need more information, we contact previous physicians and get the records.

We also look for hernias, which could be on the belly button, lower belly, or the intestines, from previous surgery.

Q: *After the nurse takes down all this information, do you meet with the patient?*

A: Yes. I think it's good for the patient to get acclimated by talking with the nurse first. When the patient comes to my office, I review the history the nurse has recorded and ask about anything that seems important. At the same time, the patient may have questions for me.

Q: *What questions do you ask the patient?*

A: It depends on the individual patient. Sometimes I don't need to ask many questions because the nurse has been extremely thorough or because the patient has volunteered a lot of information. But it is always important to get a sense as to why patients want to have liposuction, exactly what areas are bothering them, and what they expect to get out of it.

For instance, if a patient says, "I want my hips done," and the doctor looks at her hips, sees that there is some extra fat, and responds, "Fine. Go to the desk and schedule an appointment," there could be a big problem down the road. Let's say the patient expects to have five inches reduced from her hips, but there is actually only two inches of fat there. It's very important to discuss these things in detail to make sure doctor and patient are on the same page. I need to know the mind-set of the patient.

Q: *Do you ask patients how long they have been contemplating liposuction?*

A: Yes, that's a significant question. It always makes me feel better if they have been interested in it for a long time, perhaps years. Very often, they were cautious or concerned about the possible risks of the procedure. But then they saw a friend who had it done, read a story about it in the newspaper, or saw something about it on TV, and they became more interested and wanted to find out more. They see that liposuction techniques have grown and improved over the years, and they feel they are ready to try it.

Q: *So these patients are often preferable to the spur-of-the-moment types?*

A: They can be. Conservative people usually take their time to find out more about something, and by the time they come in for a consultation, they understand the procedure and their needs pretty well. Whereas someone who comes in and says, "Someone made a comment about me the other day, and now I'm tired of wearing size 14 pants and a size small top," might not have given the procedure enough thought.

Q: *Do you ask about health issues that can affect surgery?*

A: Yes. One of the most important is a patient's smoking history. Smoking is not good for many reasons, including the fact that it robs the body of oxygen. If you're smoking before or after surgery, you have an increased risk of infection and poor healing. So I ask the patients who smoke, "Do you think you will be able to cut down or eliminate cigarettes completely?"

Q: *What should patients tell you about the areas they want done?*

A: Some patients only want one area done. But others have a few areas in mind. I limit the number of areas I do in one procedure, so after we discuss the areas they want done, I may tell them, "We recommend that you have your arms, thighs, lower belly, and buttocks done. However, with the amount of fat I expect to remove and your body weight, I can only give you so much anesthetic. We can only do two of your areas safely in one session." When that happens, we may do the arms and belly for the first procedure, for example, and the next time do the buttocks and thighs.

Q: *What if patients aren't sure about what they want? What if they just feel they need some fat removed? Is that a problem?*

A: No, not usually. Some patients feel that because cosmetic surgeons have been exposed to so many different patients, they are experts and can advise them about what they need. Some might say, "Doctor, what can you do for me? I don't like my shape. Do you think it can be improved with liposuction?"

When that happens, they are giving me carte blanche. I examine them, talk to them, and then tell them what I think. For instance, "Looking at your upper back, there is fat that can be reduced with liposuction. But the fat on your belly can be reduced with dieting. The fat on your thighs will probably not go down with exercise, so we can treat that as well."

Q: *Is it important for patients to be very specific about what they want?*

A: Of course. People have individual preferences. Some like a little larger ankle or rounder buttocks, while other people want everything very flat. It is helpful to let the surgeon know what shape they prefer so the right amount of fat can be removed.

Q: *Is a person's pain threshold important?*

A: Yes. We ask them about that as well. With the tumescent liposuction I perform, we use only local anesthetic, meaning that the patients are awake during the procedure. We can give them a prescription medication to reduce anxiety if they feel they need it. But there are some patients who know themselves very well and tell us that they will not tolerate being awake for this type of procedure. They simply do not want to know what is being done. That is something I have to know in advance, because I would have to refer those people to another surgeon.

But you should also remember that tumescent liposuction is not a painful procedure. The people who do not want to be awake are usually those who become very anxious and worried and have a very low pain threshold.

Q: *Should patients discuss any previous surgeries they may have had?*

A: We do ask about that, because it gives us a sense of how they respond to surgery, how long it takes them to heal, how much bruising they may have had, and what kind of scarring they develop.

Q: *Is there any important information that patients sometimes forget?*

A: One thing that is important is whether or not they use illicit drugs. If someone is under the influence of drugs, they cannot sign a consent form with a clear head. There can also be interactions with medication we might give them. Cocaine, amphetamines, and appetite suppressants, for instance, can all interact with the anesthetic and create a dangerous load for the heart. We will not make judgments about this, but we do need to know.

Q: *Does the consultation include a discussion about the cost?*

A: It should, so if the fee has not been mentioned, the patient should ask. It might seem like common sense, but sometimes people hesitate to bring it up. It's an important piece of information. In our office, one of the staff members usually sits down with the patient to discuss it, because it's a business matter. But you should get that information at your consultation.

Q: *Can you describe the physical examination patients receive at the consultation?*

A: Patients are given a modesty garment. I examine the fat in the areas were the patient wants it removed and check its relationship to the surrounding areas.

It is important for the doctor to look at surgical scars or accidental scars, such as where you might have burned yourself on the oven, to see how they have healed. How do these scars look? What is the skin elasticity? How much fat is there between two fingers when the skin is pinched in the areas the patient wants improved? Is there any cellulite? Are there any areas of pigmentation? Is there any asymmetry? Are there any depressions or indentations in the skin? Are there potential hernias that could create a problem? Has there been gall bladder surgery, an appendectomy, or a C-section that might have created a hernia?

We also look to see how much fat they have and if the fat can be better removed through diet and exercise or by liposuction. We try to get a sense of how much time it will take to remove the fat, how much risk of getting irregularities is involved in a particular area, and whether they bruise easily.

Q: *How could you know about bruising from a physical exam?*

A: There are some women who are prone to bruising, and when they come in, they have several bruises. They are not being abused by anyone, but they bruise easily, sometimes even without contact. Some of these people have frequent headaches and take aspirin every day, and they don't realize that the blood-thinning action of the aspirin can cause bruising.

Q: *What else is discussed at the consultation?*

A: We explain the preoperative instructions patients have to follow prior to the procedure [see chapter nine]. We tell them what is likely to happen during the procedure [see chapter ten] and what happens afterward [see chapter twelve]. We want our patients to have a very clear and

complete idea of everything that is going to happen so they
won't have any unwarranted anxieties or fears about the
procedure.

Q: *How can patients get an idea of how they will look after
liposuction?*

A: I try to give them a good idea by having them look in a
mirror while I push on their fat with a few fingers so they
can see the new outline they might get. Other doctors may
use computer imaging to show patients what kinds of
results can be achieved.

Q: *But what if the surgery doesn't come out that way?*

A: This is a big concern. You can't predict results exactly, so
I don't want to give my patients any false hopes or expectations. We know that with liposuction, the fat will come
down, but we don't necessarily know how much each person's will come down. We can give patients an average.
That's why when I push on the fat while they look in the
mirror, I say, "You might get something like this," because
people heal differently.

Q: *Do you use photographs of previous patients?*

A: Yes. I show them pictures where I took out more fat than
I thought I would and pictures where I didn't get out as
much fat as I expected. It's interesting to note that sometimes

when I take out less fat than I expect to, the results can actually be better than we thought they would be. Other times, when I take out more than I expected, the patient gets less of an apparent reduction. So looking in the mirror or at photographs during the consultation only gives you an idea of the results you might get.

Q: *Should patients ask doctors about their training and experience at the consultation?*

A: Yes. They can ask how doctors learned to do liposuction, how long they have been doing it, and how many procedures they have performed. We already said that you would probably want a surgeon who has done at least 50 procedures, but if you find a surgeon who is just beginning, that surgeon might charge a reduced fee for liposuction. If you feel comfortable, you might want to consider going ahead. In general, I do think experience is important.

Q: *What should patients do if the doctor tells them they don't need liposuction?*

A: Ninety-nine times out of a hundred, it means you don't need it. If you have excess fat, you need to improve your diet and exercise program. If you don't have excess fat, you need to have a more realistic view of your body.

If a surgeon tells you don't need surgery, you can feel pretty certain that you don't need it. So what you have to do is ask the surgeon, "Why am I not a candidate for liposuction?" The doctor might say, "You're not a candidate because you are 40 pounds overweight, there's general contour fullness from your neck to your calf, and I don't know where to start and stop the procedure. You should continue with your diet and exercise and come back in six months so we can reevaluate. You should have lost 10 pounds by then. Please proceed gradually."

Q: *Are there any other reasons why a doctor would turn someone away?*

A: If I knew the patient and knew that he or she did not comply with directions, I might not want to operate. It's really important that patients follow directions very carefully in order to maximize their results and avoid medical problems.

Q: *What if you can't decide whether or not to have the surgery?*

A: The first thing you should do is try to pinpoint what's bothering you and contact the office with any further questions. If you picked a name out of the phone book and you're not happy with the physician or the office, you might want to get another name and have a second consultation.

Q: *If you and the doctor agree that you should have lipo-suction, about how long do you have to wait before you can have the procedure?*

A: That can depend on both the doctor's and the patient's schedules and other factors. A surgeon might be booked for several weeks or longer, and a patient might have to find time on his or her schedule as well. If patients are taking aspirin or certain other medications, they have to wait two weeks to get it out of their systems. Also, sometimes people have to wait until they have the payment available, because surgery has to be paid for in advance.

Q: *Can you estimate an average wait time between the consultation and the actual procedure?*

A: If patients are well informed and have decided they want liposuction by the time they come in, we can usually book them within a few weeks. But many other patients want time to think about it or to consider other options. So those patients can wait a long time before having liposuction, if they finally decide to go ahead.

POINTS TO REMEMBER

- Bring a list of your questions for the doctor to your first office visit, or consultation.

- Prospective patients must fill out several forms, including a medical history. Sometimes these forms can be obtained in advance and filled out at home.

- Patients will be asked why they want liposuction and where they would like excess fat removed.

- People who have information about liposuction and have been contemplating it for a while are often good candidates.

- If you aren't certain about where you need liposuction, the doctor can advise you.

- Sometimes patients who need liposuction on several different body areas might need to return for a second procedure.

- Patients should let the doctor know exactly how they would like each area to look following surgery.

- To protect your health, it is important to inform the doctor about any and all medications, vitamins, herbs, or street drugs you use or have recently used.

- Patients have a physical examination at the consultation so the doctor can determine if they are good candidates for liposuction.

- Some of the things the doctor looks for at the physical exam are how much excess fat you have in different areas, whether you bruise easily, how your scars heal, and how much elasticity your skin has.

- With the doctor's assistance, you can get a general idea of how you will look after liposuction, but it is not possible to know exactly.

- Some people do not need liposuction, just more dieting and exercise.

- Some people need to lose more weight before they can have liposuction and might be asked to come back in a few months following this weight loss.

- Most patients who are good candidates can schedule the surgery within a few weeks of their consultation.

7

• HOW TO MAKE YOUR DECISION

YOU'VE found a doctor you like and had your consultation. You've discussed the areas where you want to have fat removed. The doctor has given you an idea of how you will look afterward and is ready to do the liposuction procedure. But you're not sure. Liposuction is elective surgery, and you want to feel certain before you go ahead. It's a big step and a big investment.

In this chapter, we will pinpoint some of the things you should consider before you make up your mind. You definitely don't want to rush into surgery without feeling confident that liposuction is what you really want. So for most people, it's a good idea to take a little time to think about things, weigh the different factors, and wait until you feel certain about your decision before proceeding.

Q: *You mentioned the importance of feeling comfort and rapport with your physician. How important is that?*

A: I think it's very important. Cosmetic surgery is a team effort, and the members of that team are first and foremost the patient, then the physician and the staff. In cosmetic surgery, you have to make sure the physician, who has possibly never met you before, understands your desires, concerns, anxieties, and any idiosyncrasies you might have that can affect the process.

Everyone has different concerns. Some people are very anxious, and others are quite relaxed. Some people want more done than should be done, and others want less done than should be done. Some people are worried about how they will feel during the procedure, and others are worried about how they are going to look right after the procedure. So it's important that the physician gets to know enough about each patient to accommodate his or her needs.

To get the most out of this team effort, patients have to let the doctor and the staff know their preferences, concerns, and desires, and if they don't have a good rapport with the medical team, they will not be able to get these things across.

Q: *How do patient preferences affect the procedure?*

A: Some offices make efforts to accommodate each patient's needs. Patients can watch a DVD movie during surgery to keep their minds off it, if that's what they prefer.

Other people might like to wear a sleep mask because they don't want to see what is going on. Others might want to be completely involved in the procedure, and can be given a glove to feel the area being worked on. Patients should let their doctors know if they have any special preferences.

Rapport is also important after the procedure, during convalescence. If patients have concerns or questions, how will they convey them if they don't feel comfortable talking with their physician or the staff? Surgery is not just doing a procedure and walking away. It's an ongoing process, a professional relationship between the patient and the medical team.

Q: *How important are the physician's credentials, training, and experience with liposuction?*

A: These are very important considerations when making a decision about having the surgery. Liposuction is a technique that cannot be learned by reading a book, going to a lecture, or even watching someone else do it. The fundamentals need to be learned through study, but perfecting liposuction techniques can only be done through the actual experience of performing the surgery many times.

Q: *How certain should patients feel about what kind of results they will get?*

A: No one can give you a guarantee that you will have any specific amount of fat removed or any specific number of inches taken off. A physician can show you representative photographs and can demonstrate on your body how much fat is typically removed, but everyone heals differently.

Q: *So patients have to be flexible?*

A: Definitely. You have to understand that physicians will do everything they can to achieve the best results, but you still might not get that exact curve you want. Liposuction is reshaping and overall reduction in an area, but the results are influenced by many different factors, including the underlying musculature and bony framework, which is different in everyone and is also different for each body part. You can have two patients with exactly the same external measurements and remove the exact same amount of fat from the same area, and the results can be dramatically different.

Q: *In other words, you can't be 100 percent certain about your results, and you have to be able to accept that?*

A: Yes. You want to go in with realistic expectations that an area you want to be reduced will be reduced. But you can't know exactly how much it will be reduced or exactly how it will look until after the surgery.

Q: How much should you be influenced by your friends' results?

A: For many people, it gives them confidence to see that, "Okay, my friends got through it. It works. They're happy. They look good. Nothing bad happened." But again, that doesn't mean you will get the same results. So you can be positively influenced by your friends' good results, but that should never be the single deciding factor.

Q: Is it a good idea to look at before-and-after photographs in the doctor's office?

A: I think it's a very good idea, because once again, it provides you with a certain level of comfort. You see many patients who have gone through the procedure and have had very good results. On the other hand, you also have to be aware of your response to the photos. If you don't think they look good, perhaps your expectations are not realistic, or perhaps the surgeon is not as good as you would like.

The responses of prospective patients can also help a doctor understand them. If someone says, "Oh, that doesn't look so good. I want much more fat removed than that," it can let the doctor know what the patient expects and whether it is realistic.

I guess the bottom line is that if the physician shows you photos that are meant to be good examples and you don't like them, that physician might not be the right one for you.

Q: *Are there some warning signs about physicians that people should look for?* •

A: I think you have to be leery of doctors who talk in absolutes. If a physician tells you, "I have never had a problem develop in one of my patients," it can mean one of two things: Either that doctor has not done very many liposuction surgeries, or the doctor is not telling you the truth. You should also avoid physicians who, even before you have asked about the procedure, tell you that you "need" liposuction. They might correctly suggest that other areas be done along with the area you want treated to create a more aesthetic contour, but they shouldn't say you "need" the procedure. You should always understand the rationale and never feel coerced.

Q: *What can you conclude if doctors discuss possible side effects and problems they have had with patients?*

A: Every experienced surgeon has had patients with side effects, including skin irregularities such as fine crepiness or crinkles, small scars, or depressions. All surgery involves some risk, and if you are not willing to take that risk, however small it may be, you should not have elective surgery. You have to be able to deal with these problems if they happen. And of course, there are many ways for the doctor to treat these irregularities and minimize them.

Q: *What should someone considering liposuction know about possible side effects?*

A: When you decide to have liposuction, there is every possibility that you will be very happy with your surgery, recover quickly, and go back to your job and regular activities. But it might take you a little longer than you expect. You might have some persistent soreness, irregular skin tone, an indentation here or there, or some darkening of the insertion scars [see chapter thirteen]. There are many other things that can happen, and you have to be willing to accept the possibility that they might occur and you might have to deal with them.

Q: *Is it important to have exact figures on the cost of the surgery? Do you always have to pay the full amount in advance?*

A: It is very important for patients to know what the procedure costs, regardless of their income level. It's just like anything else in life. You don't want to have an unpleasant surprise. In most offices, the procedure must be paid for in full before the surgery is performed. If you need help, you can sometimes put the cost on your credit card and pay it off over time, or you can sometimes get a loan from a financing company. Some people prefer to wait until they have saved up the cost on their own. The office staff can advise you on these matters.

Q: *Should you ask the doctor what will happen if you are not satisfied with your results?*

A: You should ask, but you have to be specific about what you mean. Is it that you wanted more removed and you're not happy about that? Or do you mean that there is an asymmetry in your body after surgery? Or are you unhappy because the results are not exactly what you imagined they would be?

Surgeons can sometimes go back and remove more fat from an area if not enough was removed. Or they can remove more from one side if the results are not well balanced. But if you have your thighs done and then see that your hips also need to be done, that will be a whole new procedure that you might want to have done in the future. [See chapter fourteen for more details.]

Q: *Is it a good idea to consult family members and close friends to get their opinions? What if a close family member is against the surgery or is pressuring you to have it?*

A: Whether or not you want to consult family members and friends is a personal decision. But if a family member is cautioning you not to have liposuction, make sure you understand the reasons why. It could be that they think there's a risk involved and that you should not take a chance with an elective procedure. Or it could be that they like you the way you are and think you don't need any fat removed. If you know in your heart that you want the procedure, you should not mind explaining to your family member why you want it done and how much better you will feel afterward. Hopefully you will then get that person's support.

But if someone in your family is pressuring you to have liposuction, that is a different matter. In such a case, you should think twice about going ahead, and if you have already seen a physician and not mentioned this, you should.

The final decision has to come from deep within the patient, from their own personal feelings and beliefs and how they want to handle their own body and their own life. If they are in a relationship with someone who places a great importance on appearance, that relationship needs a lot more than some fat removal. Liposuction, or any surgery, does not fix personal problems.

Q: *If you feel uncertain about whether or not to have liposuction, how long should you give yourself to decide?*

A: As long as it takes. There is no rush.

Q: *But you've said that many patients tell you, "I wish I had done this years ago."*

A: That's true. But you should never push yourself. The time to have liposuction is when you have made up your mind and you really want it, no matter how long it takes you to come to that decision.

Q: *What if you're stuck? What if you have all the information and like the doctor, but can't make that final decision to go ahead?*

A: One thing you might do is call the doctor's office and schedule a second consultation. Bring a list of the issues that are bothering you and ask the doctor about all of them. Maybe in this discussion, the doctor can help you pinpoint what is holding you back. You might ask the doctor, "What do you think I can get out of this surgery? Are my expectations realistic? Do you feel certain I am a good candidate?"

And the doctor might ask you, "Are you concerned about the possible risks? Pain? Money? Taking time off from work? What people are going to think of you if you have cosmetic surgery?"

Once you are able to identify exactly what is troubling you, it should be easier to settle those issues.

Q: *Are there some people who should decide on no treatment at all?*

A: As I have said, no one should feel coerced into having any treatment that they do not desire themselves. Liposuction is an elective cosmetic treatment, it has some risks, and people need to be in their best physical shape, eating a well-balanced diet, and exercising regularly. Liposuction is not for everyone, and even perfect candidates might not want to undergo it for any number of reasons.

Q: *What do you say to people who think they need lipo-suction but really don't?*

A: If they are very overweight, I remind them that the pro-cedure is not a replacement for diet and exercise. If they are not overweight, I remind them that liposuction is not an appropriate treatment for people who have no excess fat to be removed. If they have psychological problems in this area, I refer them to counseling.

Some Questions to Ask Yourself Before Deciding on Liposuction

• Do I eat a basically healthy diet, or do I often binge on fatty, sugary foods that I know are not good for me and that make me put on weight?

• Do I have a regular exercise program that helps me burn calories and stay fit, and have I been following it for at least six months?

• Am I no more than 20 pounds overweight and preferably less?

• Do I have a clearly defined area of fat that will not respond to diet and exercise?

• Have I had this area for a while, or did I just gain it recently?

• Am I looking to liposuction to solve my personal prob-lems?

- Am I doing this for myself or because someone else wants me to?

- Have I found a doctor I like who has determined that I am a good candidate?

- Am I willing to follow the doctor's instructions exactly, even if they are sometimes inconvenient?

- If I am a smoker, am I willing to stop smoking for at least a few weeks, as the doctor says is necessary?

- Am I prepared to take a little time off from work and some of my regular activities?

- Am I willing to accept the results, even though they might not be exactly what I want?

- Can I afford the cost of the surgery?

- Can I deal with any possible side effects, such as soreness, bruising, or small scars?

- Will I feel better about myself if my areas of excess fat are surgically removed?

POINTS TO REMEMBER

- You should feel comfortable with your doctor, free to discuss your concerns and ask your questions.

- Make sure you are aware of your doctor's liposuction training and experience actually doing the procedure.

- You should be flexible about your results, because no one can guarantee exactly how your surgery will turn out.

- Don't use your friends' results as a deciding factor, because yours might be different.

- Looking at before-and-after photographs in the doctor's office and discussing them with the doctor can be very helpful.

- You must be prepared for possible side effects, which should be discussed with your doctor.

- Know the costs in advance, and make sure you can afford them.

- Find out what the doctor can do if you are not completely satisfied with your results.

- Have liposuction only if you want it for yourself, not just to please someone else.

- Take as much time as you need to make your decision.

- Going back to the doctor for a second consultation can often resolve issues that are bothering you and help you decide whether to go ahead.

- Overweight people who think they need liposuction might not realize that surgery is not a replacement for diet and exercise.

- People with no excess fat to remove who think they need liposuction might benefit from counseling.

For some people, the decision not to have liposuction is the best decision, especially if others are coercing them to have it and they don't really want to.

8

• THE DIFFERENT TYPES OF LIPOSUCTION PROCEDURES

YOU already know that there are several different kinds of liposuction procedures, including older methods, where you are put to sleep with general anesthesia and more modern methods, where you are awake and participating in the procedure. As with any medical field, there are new improvements coming up all the time. Before you decide to have liposuction, it is a good idea to understand something about these different approaches and make up your mind about which one appeals most to you.

Q: *What are some of the different kinds of liposuction techniques that have been used in the past?*

A: One of the first ways liposuction was done, which is no longer done today, was the "dry technique." The patient was put under general anesthesia, and no local anesthesia was used. Then the doctor would insert instruments into the fatty compartment and remove the fat with suction. What we have learned, however, is that the typical anesthetic mixture we now use, which has adrenaline in it, helps shrink blood vessels. So today, there is much less bleeding during the procedure and much less bruising afterward. With the dry technique, the blood vessels were not compressed and did not shrink, so a lot of blood was lost. Many patients even needed to have blood transfusions.

Q: *Can you review the "wet technique"?*

A: The wet technique, which means liposuction using injected fluids, was an innovation by a French surgeon, Gerald Illouz. His theory was that if he put in a solution that had a lower concentration than normal tissue fluid, the fat cells would break apart. So he developed a formula that disrupted the fat cells just enough so they could be sucked out more easily.

Q: *And when was the tumescent technique that you use developed?*

A: As previously mentioned, Dr. Jeffrey Klein developed it about 1985. But we have to clarify that there is a difference between tumescent liposuction and tumescent anesthesia. Today, there are still surgeons who put their patients to sleep with general anesthesia and who might use a modified form or genuine tumescent anesthesia for the procedure.

They are using tumescent anesthesia, but they are not performing tumescent liposuction.

Q: *What is in the tumescent anesthetic?*

A: There is a standard recipe, but physicians may change the concentration of the lidocaine. The anesthetic also contains epinephrine (also called adrenaline) in very dilute, safe dosages. The lidocaine acts as a local anesthetic and causes numbness to the surgical area; the epinephrine constricts blood vessels and decreases any bleeding during surgery. This fluid also softens tissues and makes them more responsive to surgery, because they are easier to penetrate with the cannulas.

The reason it is called "tumescent" is that the mixture fills the tissues with fluid, which then become swollen and firm. In fact, patients are sometimes amazed by how big the area gets after the tumescent anesthetic is injected.

Q: *Can you define tumescent liposuction again?*

A: Tumescent liposuction, which uses tumescent anesthesia, is surgery that is performed using only local anesthetic, with the patients awake and responsive during the procedure. It is very safe, requires only a few hours in the doctor's office, and involves minimal blood loss. Patients can go home soon after the procedure. It is quite an advance over previous techniques.

Q: *Can you define ultrasonic liposuction again?*

A: Ultrasonic liposuction employs ultrasonic machines and ultrasonic cannulas, which are the tubes that go into the fat and suck it out with a vacuum. But ultrasonic cannulas are more than just hollow tubes attached to a vacuum. They are devices that emit ultrasonic energy that heats up the tissue, which liquifies the fat. Then the machine is hooked up to a suction apparatus, and as the cannula goes to and fro, the machine vacuums out the fat the ultrasonic energy has liquified.

Q: *What is the difference between external and internal ultrasonic liposuction?*

A: The internal form of ultrasonic liposuction is what is commonly known as ultrasonic assisted liposuction (UAL). It employs a cannula that is hot, and if it's not moved back and forth or if the physician stops for a moment to think about something or check something, the hot cannula could create burn. So this procedure has greater risks.

That same hot cannula, because it is emitting so much energy, could also go through internal organs or right through the skin from one side to another. Let's say the physician is working on the left part of the belly. If the physician is not very careful, the hot cannula could go right through the skin to the right part of the belly. So internal ultrasonic liposuction requires a high level of skill, care, and concentration from the surgeon. Other possible side effects can include scarring, pigmentation, blistering, infections, and openings going into the intestine. It's a tricky procedure, and many physicians who have used it have now given it up. But some surgeons still use ultrasonic liposuction and get good results.

External ultrasonic liposuction is used to liquify fat. The ultrasonic equipment is passed over the skin and moved around with the use of a gel to avoid heating up the skin and creating a burn. Then half an hour later, the liposuction procedure is performed. If you don't use external ultrasound, you typically take out fat that has the consistency of tapioca. With external ultrasound, the fat is somewhat liquified, frothy, a much paler yellow, with a consistency of steamed milk on a cappuccino.

Q: *What are the advantages of using ultrasound for liposuction?*

A: Ultrasonic liposuction was geared for problematic procedures such as secondary procedures where there was more scarring and it was hard to go through the scar, or for the more fibrous fat that you often have with male love handles or male breasts. The idea was that the ultrasound made the movements easier on the surgeon's arm and would produce better results.

In my experience, external ultrasound breaks up and liquifies the fat to some extent, but I don't find that it makes it easier for me to do liposuction in any area or that I get better results. I use it at times, but not very often. But it is a nice, helpful way to smooth things out in the first several weeks after surgery if there is localized swelling.

Q: *You mentioned powered liposuction previously. Can you explain what that is?*

A: Powered liposuction has different forms, but they all refer to the cannula, which moves back and forth. In one type, there is a cutting blade inside the hollow cylinder. The blade turns around and cores out the fat that is pulled into the cannula, so it is a somewhat more aggressive device than those that only go back and forth quite rapidly. That allows surgeons to move their arms less, because it does more of the work for them.

For me, powered liposuction is especially helpful when I need to concentrate on a very small area of fat. I can hold the cannula in position, such as around the belly button, and it works on that small area very effectively. It's also wonderful for fibrous areas.

Q: *You also previously mentioned syringe and machine liposuction. Can you review those techniques?*

A: With syringe liposuction, a cannula is hooked up to a syringe, but these syringes are much bigger than the ones used for vaccinations, for example. The surgeon holds the syringe and pulls the plunger out, creating negative pressure or a vacuum inside the syringe. The surgeon then holds the syringe and goes back and forth to remove the fat. When the syringe is full, the surgeon gets a new one from the nurse. Some doctors are very comfortable with this procedure and use it for all their liposuction.

I prefer using the aspirator machine because I think it's cleaner and faster. I don't have to wait for the nurse to empty the filled syringe or give me a new one. Instead, my cannula is hooked up to a machine that is constantly on and the fat is going into a big bag. If the bag fills, it only takes a few seconds to change the bag and continue.

In America, the overwhelming majority of liposuction surgeons use the aspirator machine.

Q: *What is high-volume liposuction?*

A: Medical guidelines advise liposuction surgeons to limit the fat removed to not more than 4 to 5 liters per session. A liter is similar to a quart, so 4 liters is approximately 1 gallon. However, in the past, doctors were performing high-volume liposuction, removing 10 liters or more of fat at one time. When you think about the risks of general anesthesia and using it along with tumescent anesthesia, you are putting a lot of fluid into a patient in order to take out 10 liters of fat. It is really not a good idea.

Instead, the patient should be dieting and exercising, and once some of the fat is lost that way, we can use liposuction to take out the rest. At this time, we don't know if it's safe to remove more than 4 liters of fat at a time, even from an obese individual. So until we know, we do not recommend high-volume liposuction, and it is against this country's standard of care.

Q: *What is spot liposuction?*

A: That term refers to having liposuction on one little area the person doesn't like. It is a very small focus that requires only a little anesthetic. It can also be done after people have had liposuction and find one tiny area of fat remaining that they want removed.

Q: *What is full-circumference liposuction?*

A: Instead of working on the forward thighs and then coming back for the backs of the thighs, or instead of doing two areas like the inner and the front thighs and then coming back for the outer and back thighs later, a surgeon does the entire circumference. They do the fronts, the sides, and the backs all at one time. The result gives you more immediate improvement, but there is also more swelling after the surgery and a slightly greater risk of complications. But many doctors perform full-circumference liposuction with very good results.

Q: *What forms of sedation are used for liposuction?*

A: Shots can be given in the muscle to deliver narcotics and anti-anxiety medication. They can be given by mouth or injected intravenously—the choice is up to the physician and the anesthesiologist.

Q: *Are there many different sizes of cannulas?*

A: In the beginning, cannulas were 10 millimeters, which is 1 centimeter, more than a third of an inch in diameter.

Today, we're using a cannula that is much smaller, about a sixteenth of an inch. A 10 millimeter cannula is about the size of a pretzel rod. The smaller ones we use today are about the size of the smaller pretzel sticks. The size of the insertion hole relates to the size of the cannula used in that area.

The openings of the cannulas are also different. There are more aggressive cannulas to work on deeper planes when we want to get more fat out. And there are less aggressive cannulas for working on superficial planes, where we don't want to create indentations. The size we use also depends on the pattern, size, and number of the openings in the patient's skin.

Q: *Are sutures required after liposuction?*

A: True tumescent liposuction is purposely done without suturing the insertion sites. This allows an exit for the fluid, permitting it to drain out. But some doctors prefer to sew the incisions closed with sutures.

Q: *Are there scars when suturing is not used?*

A: There are scars whether stitches are used or not, but they can often be treated in the future if they bother the patients. In many cases, they are hidden, so no one sees them to begin with.

POINTS TO REMEMBER

• The dry technique, with general anesthetic and no injected fluids, had unwanted side effects and is no longer performed.

• The wet technique uses injected fluids and is very safe.

• Tumescent liposuction uses injected fluids that cause tissues to swell and allow patients to remain awake during the procedure.

• Tumescent anesthetic combines lidocaine to numb and epinephrine (adrenaline) to constrict blood vessels and minimize bleeding.

• Ultrasonic liposuction heats and liquifies fat. The internal form requires special surgical skills; the external form can be used to liquify fat prior to treatment with tumescent liposuction.

• Surgeons can remove fat with syringes or with machine-powered cannulas.

• Powered liposuction uses a high-powered cannula that moves back and forth to make fat removal faster and easier.

• High-volume liposuction, with removal of more than 4 or 5 liters of fat at one session, is not recommended.

• Different forms of sedation are available, administered by mouth or by injection.

- Cannulas come in different sizes and leave different size insertion openings.

- Some surgeons allow insertions sites to drain, while others sew them up with sutures.

9

• HOW TO PREPARE FOR LIPOSUCTION

YOU'VE done it! You've found the doctor you want, discussed your procedure in detail, given it a lot of thought, and decided to go ahead and have liposuction. You're really looking forward to finally getting rid of that annoying fat you've been trying to work off for years. The doctor's office has booked your appointment, and you want to begin preparing for the procedure. Of course, you want everything to go perfectly and you're ready to do all you can to make that happen. In this chapter, we will tell you about some of the things you can do to make your liposuction surgery a success.

Q: *Do liposuction patients need to get a medical clearance before they can have the procedure?*

A: I feel more comfortable if all my patients have a medical clearance from their primary care physicians. So yes, I do require it, but some physicians may not. I want to have the assurance that our patients are generally healthy, or at least have no medical conditions that could cause problems when they have liposuction.

Q: *Do patients need to have any pre-surgical laboratory tests to get this clearance?*

A: They do. The basic tests include a blood count, blood chemistry, and pregnancy test. It's possible that additional tests may be required by their doctors. I think that no one contemplating liposuction, regardless of their age, is immune from having an unusual medical condition, so we need to find out. That's why we require all our healthy patients to undergo this minimal testing, which includes chemistry tests to specifically make sure that they have no hidden diabetes or liver problems. We need to have the results two weeks before the liposuction procedure, just in case a test has to be repeated.

Q: *What else do you look for with these tests?*

A: We want to make sure that the electrolyte levels of calcium, sodium, and potassium, for example, are all right. If they aren't balanced, that could lead to high blood pressure, an irregular heartbeat, or other heart problems.

We use a blood count to make sure our patients are not anemic, because if they are anemic, they could be losing blood and we have to know why. We have to make sure there is no susceptibility for them to bleed easily, because that could be a major problem during and after liposuction.

We also have to make sure women are not pregnant when they have the procedure, so we do a pregnancy test on all women with childbearing potential. And we perform any other tests their general medical doctor feels are appropriate.

Any underlying condition that suppresses the immune system could be a problem. If someone has diabetes, lupus, or other immune deficiency diseases, the procedure could put them at risk. Some medications for immune deficiency diseases could also alter the lidocaine level, because both are metabolized by the liver.

There could also be hidden thyroid conditions. Let's say someone is tired or depressed a lot but just shrugs it off. If they had an undiagnosed thyroid problem, such as hyperthyroidism (an overactive thyroid gland), the adrenaline in the anesthetic could actually trigger the heart to race too much, which could have serious consequences.

We try to be as thorough as possible in making sure all our liposuction patients have no conditions, complications, or hidden health problems that could spell trouble when they have the surgery.

Q: *Are there any medications, including over-the-counter, that you should stop taking prior to liposuction, and if so, for what length of time?*

A: Our office provides detailed instructions for patients so they know exactly what to do when preparing for their surgery. We have an extensive list of medications that might increase bleeding so patients can inform the office if they are using any of them.

Some of the items that people should not take for the two weeks prior to liposuction include aspirin, vitamin E, feverfew, ginseng, gingko biloba, ginger, and garlic tablets; appetite suppressants; thyroid medication; and nasal decongestants. You also have to be careful about any medications for anxiety, fungal infections, depression, and high blood pressure, because these can interact dangerously with the anesthetic.

It's also important that patients not begin taking any new medications during this two-week period unless they let us know first. And of course, no one should ever stop taking any medication without checking first with the prescribing doctor.

Then, one week before liposuction, patients should not use any decongestants, such as Afrin Nasal Spray, Dimetapp, or Sudafed, because they can result in a dangerously high heart rate during the procedure. You should also avoid drinking more than six ounces of grapefruit juice or eating more than half a grapefruit during this week, because it can affect how the liver metabolizes the lidocaine in the anesthetic.

For the two days prior to liposuction, you should avoid certain medications, including Advil, Motrin, Ibuprofen, Nuprin, Alleve, Naprosyn, Anaprox, Feldene, and Voltaren. You must also stop taking any diet or thyroid pills, which you will discuss with the office first.

Q: *Is there a special diet that should be followed prior to surgery?*

A: You want to eat well-balanced meals with sufficient protein, because protein is needed to make collagen, and your body heals by making collagen. You should not have any alcohol for two days prior to the procedure, and you should not smoke for two weeks prior to surgery.

Q: *Are there any supplements that people* should *take prior to the procedure?*

A: Although there aren't enough scientific studies to prove its benefits, *Arnica Montana* has been taken by many people over the years and is sometimes recommended by physicians. Arnica is a herb growing in the mountains of Europe and Siberia, which is also called Wolf's bane or Leopard's bane. Anecdotal reports indicate that Arnica appears to help lessen bruising and swelling.

However, nothing is without risk. If the dose is too high, Arnica can be toxic to the heart. Until I see more definitive medical studies, I do not personally recommend Arnica for my patients.

Q: *What do people need to know about sunbathing or using tanning parlors prior to liposuction?*

A: There is no problem if you use self-tanning products before your surgery. But if you use a tanning parlor or expose your skin to the sun without protection, there is a risk of getting a burn, and if you have a burn in the area where we are doing liposuction, we can't do the surgery. The risks of an infection or the skin becoming irritated by the compression garment would be too great.

And of course as a dermatologic surgeon, I am very opposed to people using suntan parlors because of the exposure to ultraviolet rays. But if someone comes in with a tan and they are not burned, there is no reason to postpone the surgery—it won't have a negative effect.

Q: *How long should people arrange to take off from work?*

A: Realistically, three days would be fine for most people, but it depends on what you do and how rapidly you heal. At most, it should take no more than a week, but most people are back at work in three days, some in two.

Q: *Does it depend on how much physical activity you do at work?*

A: Yes, that is important. It also depends on your discomfort threshold. Some people who have liposuction on the buttocks, for instance, are comfortable sitting after three days, while others might have soreness while sitting and standing for up to two weeks.

Q: *How long should you arrange for someone to stay with you after surgery?*

A: Someone should be with the patient the night of surgery and stay through the next morning until the patient has taken a shower.

Q: *Does this person have to drive the patient home after the procedure?*

A: They can. Some people take a taxi or car service. But patients cannot drive themselves right after surgery. Someone else has to be behind the wheel. If you take a taxi or car service, you have to make sure someone is at home to meet you when you get there and remain with you until the next day.

Q: *How long do you have to be away from your regular routines, such as shopping, playing tennis, dancing, and the like?*

A: For most people, it would be about three days. But dancing might take a little longer because of the jarring up and down motion, which might hurt more than just sitting.

Q: *How long would it be before you can go on vacation?*

A: Depending on how the person is going to dress and how they look, it could be three or four days. But it's better if they don't fly for a week after surgery because changes in altitude and pressure can have an adverse effect on swelling and bruising.

When you're in a plane, there's also an increased risk of

forming blood clots because you're not moving around enough. It's a good idea not to plan a major vacation, especially one involving flying, for at least a week after the procedure.

Q: *Do patients need any special kind of clothing for the surgery?*

A: They should have loose-fitting clothing ready to put on after surgery. Big sweat pants and an extra pair of socks are recommended so patients will feel comfortable. They should also have some old sheets and towels, so in case their insertion sites are draining a little, their linen will not get stained. These can also be used for the car ride home.

Q: *Do women have to stop estrogen replacement therapy if they are still on it?*

A: If they are on it, the safest thing to do is stop at least two weeks prior to surgery. But if someone says she can't do without it, we should be able to go ahead with the procedure while she is on it. It's just important that we know about it.

Q: *What about women who take birth control pills?*

A: Informal physician polls at national meetings show that prior to performing liposuction, most physicians do not stop birth control pills unless they are the high-estrogen pills. But women should not undergo liposuction if they smoke and are on the pill, because of the increased risk of stroke with this combination.

Q: *Do people ever forget to tell you anything that's important regarding the presurgical period?*

A: People very often forget to tell us about a medication they are taking, which they take every day and have been taking for a long time. It's become so routine to them that they don't think about it anymore. But it could be really important.

Another thing people might do is take a new medication for a brief period of time for some temporary problem and then forget to tell us about it. That's also important, because certain medications remain in the system for a long time and even if discontinued or completed one day prior to surgery, they could interact with the liver and risk anesthetic toxicity.

Q: *What other things do patients have to do prior to surgery?*

A: They must purchase postoperative compression garments, which they will wear when they are swollen following surgery. They need Hibiclens or Phisoderm disinfectant, which is used to clean the skin the day before and the morning of the procedure. They must remember to fill their prescription for antibiotic pills, sedative pills, and Bactroban ointment, which should be done a week before the procedure.

POINTS TO REMEMBER

• Some surgeons require a medical clearance from your primary care physician.

• You might also need presurgical laboratory tests, including a blood count, blood chemistry, and pregnancy test.

• These tests might uncover unknown health problems that could have an impact on liposuction surgery.

• Certain medications, vitamins, herbs, and foods must be stopped prior to surgery.

• Most people need only three days off from work, although others might need more.

• Never get a sunburn prior to liposuction.

• Arrange to have someone with you the first night and the morning following your procedure.

• Remember to inform the doctor about all and any drugs you are taking or have taken recently.

• Patients need to make certain purchases prior to surgery.

• Most offices provide full written instructions for patients to follow, so nothing will be forgotten.

10

• WHAT HAPPENS DURING LIPOSUCTION

THE day has finally arrived, and you will soon be in the doctor's office to undergo your liposuction procedure. You may feel nervous or anxious about exactly what is going to happen. Will it hurt? Will it take a long time? Will you feel faint or weak? Will you be able to see the results right away? We have found that the more you know about the details of the actual liposuction procedure, the more relaxed and confident you will feel. In this chapter, we will tell you what happens during a typical liposuction procedure and answer some of the questions you might have about it.

Q: *Can you review the major areas of the body where liposuction is performed on women and men?*

A: Facial jowls and neck, upper back of the arms, upper

back underneath the bra straps, folds near the underarms, waist, love handles, hips, breast (reduction on men; some physicians also do breast reductions on women), buttocks, abdomen, belly, thighs, knees, calves, and ankles.

Q: *How is the procedure customized to suit each patient's needs?*

A: The surgeon's aim is to make the final result proportionate to that individual's contour. You don't want to create anything that looks out of place or isn't in harmony with the rest of the body. For example, you don't want the patient to look much thinner in one area than another. A good surgeon looks at each individual and figures out how to do the surgery to get the best results for that person.

We also look at the clothing they wear in the summer, when the skin is more exposed, and try to put their insertion sites in spots where they will not be visible. If a person has a particular fold or crease in the skin, we can sometimes hide the insertion site there. If someone has more fibrous, firm fat, we know we will have to work harder in those areas than on someone else, whose fat is softer. People have all kinds of special characteristics that make each procedure a little different.

Q: *What should the patient do on the day of liposuction?*

A: Take the prescribed antibiotics; eat a light breakfast with no caffeine; shower with the recommended disinfectants;

avoid moisturizer, makeup, deodorant, nail polish, and artificial nails.

Q: *Let's look at the liposuction procedure step by step. Describe what happens when the patient comes into the office on the day of surgery.*

A: We have them sign a consent form if they have not already done so and then they have an opportunity to ask questions or clarify any step of the procedure that may not be clear to them. We also give them another opportunity to ask questions right before the surgery begins. Sometimes people have been reading about liposuction the day or week before and they have some questions that haven't been answered.

Q: *What happens next?*

A: They are given a pill to alleviate anxiety, which takes about 20 to 30 minutes to take effect. Then the nurse takes the "before" photographs while the patients are wearing the same garment that they wear for the "after" photographs following liposuction. If they didn't have their measurements taken at the consultation, we take them now.

Then the nurse begins preparing the patient's skin with the disinfectant, cleaning the skin thoroughly. Before the patients arrive, the operating room has been set up with sterile sheets and a mattress warmer, which keeps them more comfortable during the procedure. After the photographs have been taken, the patient lies down on the sterile area and the nurse calls me in to the room.

Q: *What is the first thing you do when you come in?*

A: I draw lines on the patient with a marking pen to mark the areas we are going to work on. It looks sort of like a topographic map with concentric circles showing different elevations. That gives us a feeling about where the greater volume of fat is located. We might also mark areas as "no-man's-land," meaning places where we do not want to operate. We also make marks where we want to place the insertion sites.

Q: *Do you refer to the photographs while you are working?*

A: Yes. We typically have the photos printed and hung up on the wall so we can see them while we are working on the patients. Then the nurse hooks up the patients to monitors so we can check their blood pressure, heartbeat, and oxygen levels while we're doing surgery. The next thing we do is place just a little bit of local anesthetic in all the areas that will become the insertion sites. We use the smallest needle and a very slow delivery, just a tiny pinch, so the patient barely feels anything.

Q: *What do you do when the area is numb?*

A: At that point, I can make a very small nick using a larger needle with a tiny blade, through which I introduce the infiltration catheter. That is a small, long, blunt-tipped anesthetic tubing, designed with multiple openings near its end. The reason it has multiple openings is so the anesthetic can be delivered in a gentle spray rather than with a hard force.

So now the cannula is going slowly through the numbed skin into the fat, and the tumescent anesthetic slowly comes out and goes into the area we are going to work on. The patient can see this happening, they feel it happening, and the area where it is going in is now getting bigger and bigger. It is swollen with the anesthetic.

Q: *And that's why it's called tumescent?*

A: Exactly. Derived from the Latin, *tumescent* means "firmly swollen." Because the anesthetic fluid makes the area swollen and firm, the chances of bleeding and bruising are greatly decreased, making the procedure extremely safe, very much unlike the early procedures, where patients often needed blood transfusions.

Q: *What happens after the first area becomes swollen?*

A: Once the anesthetic has been placed in that area, we can proceed to numb any other areas that we might be working on, although for some patients, we might work on one area only.

Q: *How long does it take for the anesthetic to work?*

A: It usually takes at least 20 minutes for the anesthetic to have a vasoconstrictive effect, which means shrinking the blood vessels.

Q: *What do you do once the anesthetic is working?*

A: If we are working on two separate areas, I can often begin working on the first one, because the anesthetic has probably taken effect by then. We select the cannulas we want, and if we are using external ultrasound, we use it then, especially if we are working on very fibrous areas, such as the male love handles or breasts.

Q: *When does the actual fat removal begin?*

A: Now. Through the same insertion sites where I have placed the anesthetic, I now introduce the liposuction cannula. This procedure is the same whether I'm doing conventional machine-aspirated liposuction or powered liposuction.

Q: *Do you have a preference?*

A: I think powered liposuction has advantages in both fibrous and conventional areas. One reason is its vibrational effect. It seems to distract the patients, and they also don't seem to feel as much with the rapid to and fro of the cannula. Many patients describe it as something like getting hummed to sleep, with their bodies being rocked with little vibrations, lulling them into a very relaxed state. And patients who have experienced both types tell us that they like the powered liposuction more.

Q: *How do you know where the fat is and how much to remove?*

A: In general, that is something you learn from experience. When I perform liposuction, I'm using both my hands. My left hand, which is called the "brain hand," is guiding the procedure, feeling where the tip of the cannula is and helping guide it to the fat. Sometimes, when the fat is not coming out easily, the brain hand can guide the fat to the cannula.

My right or dominant hand is holding the cannula as it goes back and forth and suctions out the fat. You get a sense when you are within the areas that have been anesthetized, and you know you are above the muscle wall, not too close to the bone, not too close to the skin, and within the fat you want to get out. It's difficult to describe to someone who has not actually done it.

Q: *What else is going on as the fat is removed?*

A: I start in the deeper plane of fat and then move up to a higher plane and so on, because I'm working in a three-dimensional area. If I work vertically at first, then I do the same thing horizontally. I repeat this procedure through all the insertions sites that have been marked.

Q: *Do you use different cannulas?*

A: Yes. I almost always change the size of the cannulas. There are different theories about whether you should go from smaller ones to bigger ones or vice versa. In most cases, I work from a smaller cannula to a bigger one, which I find more effective in creating tunnels to remove the fat. It also creates less discomfort for the patients in case the area isn't completely numb.

Q: *What is happening to the patient's body as you work?*

A: Gradually, the area that we're working on is diminishing, the volume of fat is going down, and we are contouring and tapering it so there will be no obvious border between the area that was treated and the area next to it that was not treated.

Q: *How do you monitor your patients?*

A: As we're working, we're also checking to see how the patient is doing. We constantly speak with them, check their facial expressions, see how they are reacting, and make sure they are comfortable.

Q: *What can you tell from the appearance of the fat as it's coming out?*

A: We examine the fat as we do the procedure. If we've been working in one area for a little while and we start to see the fat turning a little less bright yellow and a little more toward pink, then we know we are getting a little bleeding and we need to move on to the next area. So we're not only looking at the patients and the shape of their bodies, we're also looking at the fat that's being removed.

Q: *What about symmetry?*

A: That's very important. We use our notes and preoperative pictures to guide us. We know that if someone was much heavier on the right side, we have to take out more fat on the right side, if possible, to even things up.

Q: *What happens when you have removed as much fat as you can?*

A: At that point, I tell the patients that we are going to sit them up and then stand them up. We give them time until their blood pressure equilibrates and then help them slowly sit up. The nurse is always right by their side and helps them stand, in case they feel a little lightheaded from lying down for so long. Then we help milk out some of the fluids with a gentle massage.

The next thing is to look at and feel the body to see how much has come down. We try to find out if there is more left that can be removed, or if one area is a little more lumpy than the other. We run our hands across the area and perhaps say, "Oh, here's a tiny lump. Let's go ahead and work on this spot a little more."

Q: *Can the patients also see what has been done so far?*

A: Yes. They get to see the results immediately, which is a very big advantage of tumescent liposuction. The patients are awake and can interact with the surgeon and the staff and let us know how they feel about what is going on. They can stand up immediately, and we can all see what residual fat is there, if any, so it can be taken out.

Q: *So they can have a pretty good idea of how they will look later on?*

A: They have an idea, but it isn't exact because the anesthetic makes the skin look different. It's swollen and plumper, and it's also paler in color. And the skin surrounding the area we've worked on can look more fatty, swollen, dimpled, and cellulitelike than it did before and than it will after they heal. We have to point that out and remind them that it is not going to look this way later on.

Q: *What happens when the surgical part of the procedure is over?*

A: Once we are convinced we are finished with the surgery, the nurses clean up the patients and because there is still fluid oozing out of the insertion sites, the nurses give them fresh sheets to lie on. We dress the little insertion sites without stitches, putting some antibiotic ointment on them and then some sterile tape, allowing the fluid to continue to come out, which is a safety feature of the procedure.

Then we give our patients some refreshments, which is typically a platter of fresh fruit. After that, the nurse helps them put on the compression garment, which is an extremely important part of the procedure. The nurse explains how to put on the garment properly and how to put on further dressings to help absorb the oozing fluids that may continue to come out for a while and then helps them get dressed.

Q: *What sensations do patients feel while the liposuction procedure is going on?*

A: The most common reaction we get is, "Oh, I can't believe I waited so long to have it. This is nothing. This is great." They can't believe that they are not having any real pain. When the anesthetic goes in, they might say, "That feels cool," or sometimes, "It's stinging a little bit," which is a clue that I need to slow down the rate at which the anesthetic is being delivered.

With tumescent liposuction, the patients communicate with us throughout the procedure. So if they feel even the slightest discomfort, we can adjust what we are doing immediately. If they say "Ouch," while we are putting in the anesthetic, we instantly slow down the rate of delivery and they are fine. If we hit a sensitive area while we are removing fat and they say "Oooh," or "Ow," we can put a little more anesthetic there and perhaps enter the area from a different direction, or go on to another area and then come back later.

There are certain areas that are more sensitive than others, such as the belly button, which can be very tender. I take time to numb those areas. If you're doing liposuction in the abdomen, you might rub up near the rib cage or the diaphragm, so those areas also have to be numbed carefully.

The hip bone is also a tender area, and when we're working there, the cannula could bump up against it and there could be a little discomfort for a fraction of a second.

Toward the end of the procedure, when we want to smooth things out, patients might start to feel a little more as the anesthetic is wearing off a bit.

Overall, people tend to describe liposuction as a cool sensation, maybe slightly stinging as the anesthetic goes in, but not bad at all, something like a massage. For the most part, they are just lying there watching television or a video or listening to music and feeling a slight tingling every now and then. In most cases, they tell us, "I can't believe that this is all that's involved with it." Sometimes they're even telling us jokes and we're telling them jokes.

Q: *What is the difference between the tumescent procedure you have described and liposuction with general anesthetic?*

A: The differences are that with general anesthetic, the patient is asleep and can't respond to the procedure as it is being done. The surgery might be quicker because the surgeon doesn't have to worry about hurting the patient. And the surgeon might not be able to use all the fluids we use in the tumescent procedure, so there could be more bruising and pain after surgery. Patients also take longer to recover and return to full function, so they can't immediately go to the bathroom, get dressed, or go home. Some of them may feel sick from the general anesthesia. They can also wake up colder from general anesthesia once it wears off. Tumescent anesthesia lasts longer.

Q: *How long does the tumescent anesthetic last?*

A: It can remain in the blood for about 12 to 16 hours. The area is numb for only about four to six hours in some patients.

Q: *Approximately how many incisions are made during a procedure?*

A: If it's a central area, like the belly or neck, it's usually only two or three. If it's a procedure that has to be done on two sides, like the hips, each side might have three separate insertion sites. The average is two or three per area, but they can go up to as many as five per area. In my practice, the largest number someone might have with one day of liposuction would be approximately 12 insertion sites, but the average is well under that, more like 6 or 8 at most.

Q: *About how much fat is typically removed?*

A: Probably the smallest amount is about 25 ccs of fat, which would be from an area like the inner knees. The neck might be between 50 and 75 ccs. And although the standard of care is not to remove more than 4 to 5 liters of fat, I typically do not remove more than 3 liters of fat, and more likely it is somewhere between 1 and 2 liters.

Q: *How does that translate into pounds?*

A: A recent survey found the typical weight loss from liposuction is 5 to 7 pounds. Because I am not as aggressive as some other surgeons, my patients probably lose from 2 to 5 pounds. But for many people, it's the inches that really count, and sometimes, depending on where the liposuction is performed, they may go down a full dress size or even two.

Q: *What are some areas of the body that are often combined in one procedure?*

A: Typical combinations are the neck and jowls, the upper back and underarm folds, the waist and the abdomen, the waist and the outer thighs, and the buttocks and the outer thighs. Another grouping is the inner thighs and the inner knees. Because I do more thighs, I might do the outer and front thighs in one session and the backs of the thighs and inner thighs in another session.

Q: *Do you recommend combining liposuction with other cosmetic surgical treatments, such as face-lifts or breast implants?*

A: If the liposuction procedure is a small one, let's say liposuction of the neck, it might be appropriate for the surgeon to do a neck-lift at the same time. Aside from that, I don't recommend it, mainly because of the risks when other cutting procedures are done at the same time. There could be a risk of anesthetizing patients for too long a period of time, and there is also an increased risk of infection by having open wounds in too many different places. Also, this is when serious complications have occurred.

Q: *How long does a patient have to be in the doctor's office for a typical tumescent liposuction procedure?*

A: From walking in the door to leaving the office, it is usually about four to five hours. It's about half an hour from the time they go into the room and sign the consent, have photos taken, and have their skin prepared. Then it's about another 30 minutes before they are ready for me to enter the operating room. Then the marking and discussion could take another 10 to 15 minutes. It can take a half hour to an hour to put in the anesthetic, depending on how many areas we will be doing. Then it can take from 15 minutes to 1 hour to do the actual liposuction on each area. When we're finished, it takes about 10 minutes for refreshments, then about half an hour to clean up, put on the garment, and review the instructions. I'd estimate that the average patients are in the office for four or five hours.

POINTS TO REMEMBER

- Liposuction surgeons carefully assess each patient's needs and then individualize the procedure to meet those needs.

- When you know exactly what to expect during the liposuction procedure, you will probably not have any fear or anxiety.

- Tumescent liposuction patients remain awake during the procedure and can communicate easily with the medical team.

- Most patients are surprised at how comfortable they feel during the procedure and often wonder why they waited so long to have it.

- Tumescent liposuction patients can sit or stand after fat removal and can help the doctor determine if there is any additional fat that needs to be removed.

- Because of swelling, patients can't see the exact results they will have until after some time has passed.

- Some patients might feel slight discomfort for a few seconds during the procedure, but they can inform the doctor, who will immediately take care of any problems.

- For most body areas, two or three incisions are used at most. The average patient has a total of approximately six to eight incisions.

- Average patients lose between two and seven pounds.

- At times, liposuction can be combined with other cosmetic surgical procedures.

- A typical patient is in the doctor's office for liposuction between four and five hours.

11

• HOW LIPOSUCTION CAN REDUCE DIFFERENT BODY AREAS

YOU already know that the liposuction procedure and results are different for each individual and can be influenced by many different factors. Perhaps you have only one small bulge of fat that you have been unable to get off with diet or exercise. Or perhaps you have three or four areas where excess fat bothers you. No matter what your situation, you are naturally curious about what liposuction can do in that specific area of your body. In this chapter, we will give you a general idea of how surgeons work in each body area, exactly what is done to remove the fat, and what kind of results you might be able to achieve.

Q: *When doctors learn to perform liposuction, are they trained to do it on every body part?*

A: Liposuction training is more universal, and surgeons do not receive any special training for each part of the body. We learn to do each body part through actual experience, so it makes sense for patients to ask surgeons how many procedures they have done on the part of the body that the patients want treated.

Q: *What if the surgeon's experience on that part is limited?*

A: Patients could take that into account. However, the surgeon might be very accomplished, and the patient might feel a lot of confidence in that doctor. Good surgeons also know their limitations. This is something you have to discuss and work out with your surgeon on an individual basis.

Facial Jowls and Neck

Q: *What are the jowls?*

A: Some people may have just the beginning of some sagging right underneath their jaw line. The jowls are the little fat pads that come on the forward part of the jaw and hang down over the jaw. When you're looking straight at a person with jowls, you see a little sagging fat coming down to the neck, over the jaw, between the chin and the middle part of the jaw.

Q: *What causes that?*

A: Jowls are thought to be related to some kind of thinning or weakening of the supporting elastic tissue that occurs with time and gravity, but it hasn't been very well studied.

Q: *What can liposuction do for the facial jowls?*

A: If someone has a little sagging there and doesn't want to have a full or mini-face-lift, liposuction can often remove enough fat to get some flattening of the jowls.

Q: *What can liposuction do to change necks?*

A: We hope that by now people will realize that just because they have a double neck or a low-lying neck, that doesn't necessarily mean liposuction can improve it. There has to be excess fat. If your neck is not really composed of an excess amount of fat, then liposuction won't help much.

Q: *Who is the ideal candidate for liposuction of the facial jowls and neck?*

A: The ideal candidate is somebody who is not ready for a face-lift and just has a minimal to moderate amount of fat hanging over the jaw on to the neck. Ideally, there should be no extra skin that has to be pulled up. For people like this, liposuction with minimal incisions can create a nice angle of the neck.

Q: *Is liposuction an alternative to a face-lift?*

A: No. The surgeon has to examine the patients and tell them what they need. Sometimes patients need both. They can have some liposuction of the neck and the jowls and then have a lift to remove the sagging. Other people need only a lift because they don't have any excess fat, and removing the fat they have would only thin out the area and make them look gaunt. Other people need only liposuction, because they don't have any extra skin, only excess fat.

Q: *Is there a way people can figure out what they need on their own?*

A: If someone is looking at their neck and they don't like it, they can pinch the skin between two fingers and make what we call a "frog neck." They tighten up the platysma muscle, which is between the collarbone and the chin. When they do that, if they are able to pinch a bulky amount between the muscle and the skin, that is a sign that, in all likelihood, some fat can be removed with liposuction.

Q: *What do you mean by a "frog neck"?*

A: Rest your hands on the skin of your neck and then make a grimace to tighten that neck muscle. You should feel the muscle pulling up high, as if it's pulling on the collarbone.

Q: *What is the typical age range for people who have these procedures?*

A: Typically, patients' jowls start to form in their 50s. With the neck, it can start rather young, especially if it's an inherited tendency. People as young as their 20s have had neck-lifts.

Q: *Is there anything special surgeons evaluate for the jowls and neck?*

A: Some people have a very low Adam's apple, and the angle of their neck can never be as sharp as someone with a higher Adam's apple. People with low Adam's apples will not get the same results, and that has to be taken into account when preparing for surgery.

Q: *Approximately how long does surgery for the neck and facial jowls take?*

A: It can take between 20 and 40 minutes for the actual liposuction, but the preparation and post-surgical treatment also take time, as we have seen. In all, they might be in the doctor's office for around two hours.

Q: *How many incisions are needed, and where are they placed?*

A: Between one and three incisions are placed underneath the chin and underneath the earlobes.

Q: *Does surgery in this area feel different in any way?*

A: Swelling in the neck does feel different from other body parts. People describe it as a "strange" feeling, but remember that it is only the outer part of the neck, the compartment above the muscles, that swells. There is no swelling of the inner neck or airway, so there is no effect on swallowing, for instance. It might feel weird, but there is no discomfort or pain.

Q: *How long is the convalescence?*

A: Patients can be at home for a day or two and then go out, as long as they don't mind wearing a chin-strap garment in public.

Q: *How long is the healing process?*

A: The insertions sites usually heal in two days, and bruising is gone in one or two, or rarely three, weeks. The swelling will last a little longer, but the compression chin-strap garment will help that.

Q: *How long do people have to wear the chin strap?*

A: It is best to wear it all the time for at least two weeks and for an additional two weeks at night. Some patients prefer to have tape compression for their necks so they look less obvious.

Q: *How does the typical patient look when everything has healed?*

A: Much better! Typically, there is an immediate improvement. On the neck, in contrast to some other areas, the thinning that has been done with liposuction is significant and can be easily seen. But because there is swelling for a few days, you don't get the full effect right away. Sometimes there are minor temporary side effects such as indentations from the chin strap or some crepiness or fine lines under the chin, but for almost everyone, those lines improve a great deal over the first few months. In the best cases, patients look like they had a face-lift.

Q: *So other people really notice?*

A: They notice something is different, but they don't usually realize what it is. They may say, "Were you on vacation?" or "Did you lose weight?" or "Is that a new haircut?" They know something is different and they know the person looks a lot better, but often they have no idea that any kind of surgery was involved.

Arms

Q: *Which patients are good candidates for arm liposuction?*

A: Patients who tend to have not just loose skin that is sometimes hanging and of poor quality, but those who have actual fat in the back of the upper arm are good candidates. Although the forward arm can be done, the most common area for liposuction is the back of the upper arm. The skin should have some elasticity. If not, it might be necessary to have surgery to remove some of the skin afterward. We do the liposuction first and see how it heals. Most patients who have this surgery are in their late 40s and older. Younger patients often get good results with liposuction alone.

Q: *Are these patients mostly women?*

A: Yes, although I have seen men who could benefit from it. Because of how fat accumulates in women, they are much more likely to undergo the procedure on their arms.

Q: *How does the surgeon evaluate your arms?*

A: I use two positions: with arms outstretched to the sides and then with elbows bent at a right angle so the hands are going straight up to the ceiling. When their arms are outstretched, I pinch the skin of the upper back of the arm between my fingers and feel the amount of fat there. Then I have them flex their elbow and push against my hand, trying to extend their arm out straight. This tightens the triceps muscle, and pinching the skin reveals the fat above the muscle. I can get a sense about whether there is excess fat and if they will get a good result from liposuction, depending on the shape of the underlying muscle and how much loose skin they have.

Q: *Approximately how long does this surgery take?*

A: They need to be in the office for three to four hours. The actual liposuction surgery takes from two to two and a half hours.

Q: *How many incisions are needed, and where are they placed?*

A: There are at least three incisions placed near the underarm, near the elbow, and midway up the upper arm.

Q: *How does this surgery feel to the patient?*

A: After the anesthetic goes in, it feels swollen and tight. Because patients are lying down with their arms straight out, there can be a feeling of "pins and needles," so we try to have them change position every now and then. Once the arms are numb, the patients feel a back-and-forth massage, and if we're doing powered liposuction, it can feel like a soothing vibratory massage. There is usually no discomfort or pain.

Q: *Is a compression garment needed after surgery?*

A: Some physicians require them only for a few days, but I find that the garments make most of my patients feel more comfortable, so I have them wear the garments for 24 hours a day for about 2 weeks, then at night for another 2 weeks.

Q: *How long do patients have to be away from work?*

A: It depends. If you don't use your arms too much at work, you can go back in two to three days. If you use your arms for manual labor, you can go back in at least one week and probably two. For those first two weeks, the arms will be pretty tender. But you certainly can do all the things you normally do at home, such as dress, prepare meals, and feed yourself. It might feel a little tight because of the garment, so you have less agility, but you can do everything a bit more slowly and deliberately.

Q: *Are women who have had mastectomies good candidates?*

A: If a woman has had a mastectomy and also had her lymph nodes under her arms removed, she may be susceptible to chronic swelling. This could be exacerbated by liposuction, and there could be serious complications, including infections. Therefore, I would be very reluctant to work on such a patient, and if I were to consider it, I would need approval by the surgical oncologist who removed the lymph nodes.

Q: *What would the ideal results of this surgery be?*

A: A perfect result would be that the patient's skin has great elasticity and there would be a little fat left to act as an insulator. You would have a subtle outlining of the arm muscles. Your arm would look thinner but not too thin, and there would be no loose hanging skin and no rippling or indentations, just nice muscle definition and a pleasing appearance.

There is significant improvement in most patients, but not every patient gets the precise results they want. The volume of fat will definitely decrease, but for some patients, the percentage of improvement might not be as great as they wanted.

Breasts

Q: *In the chapter on men (chapter sixteen), we will discuss using liposuction for breast reduction, which is a commonly performed procedure. What about breast reduction in women?*

A: There are liposuction surgeons who are doing mini-breast reduction in women, but I am not one of them. I say "mini" because if a woman's breasts are very large, low, heavy, and causing pain in the back and the grooves of the shoulders from bra straps, chances are that liposuction will not be enough to correct it. Furthermore, as the breasts age, the position of the nipples gets lower on the chest.

Liposuction of the breast, which reduces the girth of the breast, does not necessarily change the nipple position. A true breast reduction not only reduces the amount of fat in the breast, but it also repositions the nipple. So you have to have the right candidate and the right physician, one who thoroughly understands every aspect of breast surgery.

There is also a concern about complications that could compromise the patient's medical health. Could liposuction of the breast result in scar tissue or calcification that might affect the results of a mammogram? These considerations give me pause, and I am not yet convinced that using liposuction for breast reduction in women is completely sound.

Q: *What do you currently tell patients about your views on liposuction for breast reduction in women?*

A: I explain that liposuction of the breast for mini-reduction is still investigational and I think potential patients should follow future findings and feel completely certain it is safe before they have it done.

Q: *But there are liposuction surgeons who perform this procedure?*

A: Yes. There might be cosmetic surgeons and plastic surgeons who do it, but I have no information on how many there are.

The Upper Back

Q: *What kind of liposuction is performed on the upper back?*

A: This surgery is typically performed on women. There are a couple folds that occur when increased fat accumulates in the upper back. They are right behind the underarm, and parallel folds underneath the bra strap area. These areas are amenable to treatment.

Q: *Many people try to lose that fat by working out, don't they?*

A: Yes, but working out in the gym, doing push-ups or sit-ups, and using those muscles a lot does not increase the activity level of the fat in the vicinity. Just because you are using a muscle that is located underneath an area of fat that you want to reduce, that doesn't mean the activity will actually reduce the fat.

Q: *Can you describe a typical patient for upper back liposuction?*

A: Many times, these women are in their mid-50s, not at their ideal body weight, and unable to reduce further. They are usually uncomfortable in clothing because their excess fat is bulging through their clothes. So when we do liposuction, we work on the rolls of fat we want to reduce. Of course, we first have to determine if the rolls are actually fat or if they are just sagging skin folds. Unfortunately, it is sometimes impossible to make the rolls that push out under or over the bra straps disappear completely.

Q: *How long does the surgery take?*

A: The time for the surgery depends on how many rolls of fat we have to reduce. The average procedure takes about one and a half to two hours, so patients have to be in the office for about four and a half hours.

Q: *What about the insertion sites?*

A: There are several, depending on how many rolls need to be reduced. They might be located along the midline near the spine and on the borders between the sides of the chest and the back, such as underneath the arm.

Q: *What kind of results can be achieved?*

A: Liposuction is very helpful for some women, and they show a lot of improvement; but for others, it is not as effective. That's why we are very careful during the consultation to try to determine who will get good results. Do they have enough fat that is going to come out to make the rolls reduce? Women who have a significant amount of fat in those rolls stand to have considerable improvement.

Q: *Does the back ever end up completely flat?*

A: You cannot realistically expect everything on the back to be totally flat, especially with a bra strap pressing in on the skin. But you will get an improvement in terms of how patients look in clothing and how they feel about themselves.

Flanks

Q: *Can you explain what the flanks are?*

A: They are the sides of the body between the underarms and the hips.

Q: *How can liposuction help in this area?*

A: There are people who have a mound of fat that begins somewhere a few inches below the underarm and then comes down before the waist really starts, extending from the back part of the side of the chest and going around to midway between the spine and side of the chest. In men, the love handles are considered the flanks. The flanks respond very nicely to liposuction.

Q: *How do you assess these patients?*

A: We have to look at where the waist starts, because we want an even flow from one area to another. We don't want an abrupt transition from the flank to the waist or hip. We are looking for a subtle reduction in volume, ending up with a nice smooth contour between the different parts of the body.

Q: *Is there anything special about the surgery?*

A: The flank area in some women consists of more fibrous fat, so you have to work slowly when you are liposuctioning there. Also, the ribs are right underneath, and you want to be careful not to rub the cannula too close to the bones. But if you use slow, deliberate strokes, it should be a rather easy procedure.

Q: *What happens after surgery?*

A: The garment for the flank area is usually the same as a chest garment. But there are times when we need to use an abdominal binder as well to reinforce the lower part. It's like a corset, going around in a circle and fastening at the back with Velcro.

Waist and Hips

Q: *How is liposuction done on the waist and hips?*

A: You can work on the waist at the same time you work on the flanks. You want to get an even flow from one to the other. In women, you don't want to create a masculine V-shape torso, so when you work on the waist, you can use some of the same incisions you use for the flanks. Because of the curvature of the waist, it's hard to use lower insertion areas, such as around the hips.

The anterior approach to the waist can be done at the same time as liposuction on the belly (see below).

Right below the waist are the hips, which can be treated from the back and the front. We put insertion sites a couple inches away from the spinal column, as well as on the sides of the chest, so we can approach from above. The surgery is done both vertically and horizontally. There are usually three insertion sites per side.

Q: *Is it risky to work so close to the spine?*

A: Many patients are concerned about that, but it is safe because we are still far away from any nerves and there is also a layer of muscle between the spine and the fat.

Abdomen and Belly

Q: *What do you look for when evaluating a patient for lipo-suction on the abdomen?*

A: Once again, the first thing we look at is whether the patient is a good candidate. Will they get good improvement because their muscles are strong and they have excess fat that needs to be removed? Sometimes we find that the bulge we see is actually a condition called "diastasis," where the muscle is not supported and is pushing forward. In these cases, there is often minimal fat above the muscle wall and the bulge is not really fat, so liposuction would not be helpful.

Q: *What about the belly?*

A: Again, we have to be certain that there is a need to remove fat and that the extra bulge of the belly is not caused by hanging skin. Sometimes, people need a tummy tuck or other forms of surgery on the abdomen and belly. Sometimes, both liposuction and a tummy tuck are the best option.

Q: *Are a tummy tuck and liposuction done at the same time?*

A: It is much safer to do them in separate procedures to avoid the possibility of a fat embolus, which is a traveling particle of fat that can create dangerous complications if it reaches the heart, lungs, or brain. This complication is not seen when tumescent liposuction is done alone, so liposuction is usually done first and then the patient can have the tummy tuck later on.

Q: *What are some of the things you have to consider during abdominal liposuction?*

A: You have to determine whether you are dealing with the whole abdomen or the upper and lower areas, and if the area is heavy with fat. This is one of the typical areas where women store extra fat, and the removal has to be done very carefully to avoid an imbalance in the results.

Q: What about the belly procedure?

A: Patients have to realize that gravity pulls the liposuction fluids down, so within a day or two after the procedure, some women find that the labia around the vagina are very swollen, while men might find their scrotum swollen. These areas can also be bruised, which can frighten patients if they are not told about it in advance and know what to expect.

Most often, the fat here is soft, especially in the lower belly. Most people have a little mound of fat that comes out with minimal effort.

Q: Is this swelling painful?

A: No, it's just uncomfortable. You might not be able to do your normal exercise routine for a few days.

Q: Are there special considerations for the belly button area?

A: Similar to the ribs, the belly button is a very sensitive area. We have to make sure it is completely numb before we begin working.

Buttocks

Q: *What are the special considerations for working on the buttocks?*

A: This is a challenging area, because each person has a different idea of how he or she wants the area to look after surgery. Of course, you can't always get the precise results patients want. Just the right amount of fat has to be removed, which is not always easy.

For some people, the fat is in the upper buttock, and for others, it's in the upper outer buttock or the lower outer buttock. The upper outer buttock goes along with the waist, and the lower outer buttock coincides with the outer thighs. So you have to be aware of the contour you want to achieve.

Q: *How much reduction can you get?*

A: It can be significant, but just because you remove a lot of fat, that doesn't necessarily mean that the result will be aesthetically pleasing. For example, there are different ligaments that help hold the buttocks in place, and sometimes the buttocks can fall or create new bulges or new creases. A surgeon has to be aware of all these different factors.

Q: *Are there any special circumstances involved with buttock liposuction?*

A: Some patients have a significant amount of fat in the inner lower quadrants and not much in the outer areas of the buttocks. Only a conservative amount of fat should be removed to avoid a flattening of this area. The crease under the buttocks should be avoided. The area of the upper back thigh under the buttock, which often protrudes, must be suctioned superficially to avoid weakening the support. Otherwise, the buttock may drop and create a second crease, forming a "banana fold" (a horizontal mound of fat between the two creases).

Q: *Who are good candidates?*

A: Once again, it's people who have worked for a number of years, through diet and exercise, but can't get rid of that bulge of fat on the buttocks. For these people, liposuction is a wonderful treatment. Buttock liposuction can help reduce the overall circumference so clothes fit much better.

Q: *How long is a typical procedure?*

A: About two and a half hours, with patients in the office for four to five hours.

Q: *What about convalescence?*

A: Patients wear garments for 24 hours for the first two weeks, and then for another two to four weeks at night. They might be sore for a few weeks, and it might be uncomfortable to sit for long periods of time. Again, it depends on the individual. Some people heal very quickly.

Thighs

Q: *Do many people have liposuction on the thighs?*

A: Similar to the belly, the thigh area is very commonly done. Many women have inherited a tendency to develop deposits of fat in their outer thighs that they cannot reduce, no matter how much exercise and dieting they do. Often, they have had this condition since adolescence or early adulthood and have really tried to watch their weight and exercise regularly, but it just won't go away. This area is commonly referred to as "saddlebags," and many women in their 30s are now coming in to have them done.

But women through their 50s, in all different shapes and sizes, suffer from this problem. Some have more fat on one side than the other, and we try to even it out as we remove the fat.

Q: *Are there any special problems in working on the thighs?*

A: It is not always possible to make things exactly symmetrical when the thighs are not the same size to begin with. Some people have more bony prominences, and their results might not be the same as their friends' because of that.

The thighs are also an area where cellulite is commonly found, and as we know, cellulite does not usually improve with liposuction. There can be a deep depression over the head of the thighbone (femur) at the hip if there is too much fat removed at this point. The inner thigh tends to create sagging folds and irregularities more than any other area, and this area must be approached conservatively. Sometimes it is not possible to safely remove enough fat to achieve a good result.

Q: *Who are ideal candidates?*

A: The best candidates are people who are relatively young and very near their ideal body weight or just slightly above and who can't remove that last bulge on their outer thighs with diet and exercise.

Q: *Where are the insertion sites?*

A: There are usually one or two along the waistline, and others may be in the crease between the buttock and thigh and below the outer thigh closer to the knee. If we are doing the thighs at the same time as the buttocks, we can sometimes get to the thighs through at least one of the buttock insertion sites.

Q: *Is there a lot of bruising from this procedure?*

A: There is always some bruising, but it has been much less with tumescent liposuction than the earlier forms of this surgery. That's why compression garments are important during the healing process.

Q: *How long does this surgery take?*

A: It varies, according to the amount of fat that has to be removed and where it is. Generally, liposuction on the thighs takes from one to three hours, requiring someone to be in the office for three to five hours.

Q: *What does the surgery feel like to the patient?*

A: Sometimes the fat is more fibrous in this area, and in those cases, it feels like a vigorous massage. It is usually not painful, but it can feel a little sore while we are doing it, especially toward the end of the procedure as we're getting out the last of the fat. If that happens, more anesthetic is given immediately.

Q: *What kinds of results can people expect?*

A: The thighs are an area where many women derive significant reduction, and they can see it right away in how their clothing fits. However, it might not be as evident when you look at the thighs. For example, if a liter of fat is removed from the outer thighs of some women, the before-and-after pictures might not show that much of a difference. But in other women, you can remove half that amount and because the area is smaller and more defined, you will see a definite change in contour from the hip to the knee.

Q: How long does it take to recover?

A: Most people are back at work in three days and back in the gym in one to three weeks. As with all liposuction procedures, each person responds differently.

Q: Is there any way people can figure out if they are good candidates?

A: There are some people who do not have excess fat in the thighs at all but think they do. It's actually the outer buttocks pushing down and it's the buttocks that need treatment. These are called "pseudo saddlebags," and it is possible for people to check this themselves at home.

You need two mirrors so you can see your rear without turning your head around. Clench your buttocks firmly and tighten them up. If you see that your outer thigh goes in by a half inch to an inch, your buttocks are probably contributing to the fatty appearance of your thighs. And if your thighs look perfect when you clench your buttocks, you might want to think about having liposuction on your buttocks, not only your thighs.

Knees

Q: Who would benefit from liposuction on the knees?

A: Knees are often requested by women who complain that they feel their knees rubbing together when they walk. Many dancers are terribly bothered by this, as well as models who dress in skirts and shorts. There could be many reasons for this rubbing, including an extra fat pad on the inner knee or an unusual orthopedic condition because of the way their hips are constructed. No matter what the reason, when there is extra fat on the knees, we can remove it through two very small insertion sites, one below the area in the inner knee and the other in the back where the crease is behind the knee.

Q: *How long does this procedure take?*

A: In a very fast procedure, it could take 10 minutes to numb both areas, 30 minutes for the anesthetic to take effect, and perhaps another 15 to 20 minutes to remove the fat from both knees. Many times, the knees are done along with the inner thighs or outer thighs. Afterward, we put on compression tape and sometimes use a full compression garment.

Q: *How much fat can be removed from the knees?*

A: Typically not much fat is removed, but it is enough to resolve the problem, and most people are very happy with the results.

Q: *What about healing?*

A: There is usually a bit of bruising and swelling, but the knee doesn't swell as much as other areas of the body.

Then, after a few weeks of compression, the knees look really good.

Calves and Ankles

Q: *What kind of results can you get with liposuction on your calves and ankles?*

A: You get volume reduction, rather than a large change in contour, so the girth is decreased, but it might not result in a large change when you look at it. There is not much fat in the calf or ankle. The result can be a subtle, but dramatic, reshaping of the inner and outer profiles of the lower legs when you look straight at the legs. You can get better muscle definition in the calf, but most women are not looking for that. Some ankles are so large that they give the impression of stumps. Once there is better definition of the Achilles tendon and ankle bones, the legs have a more tapered silhouette.

Fatty calves and ankles are often an inherited condition that patients have had from childhood, even when they have no weight problems. So when they are able to get rid of this fat, they are usually very happy.

Q: *In what other ways is surgery on these areas different?*

A: There is typically a lot of swelling when you do liposuction on the lower legs. The lower legs take much longer to heal than the face because of body circulation and gravity. So although swelling on the thigh or belly might be totally gone in a few weeks, swelling on the calves or ankles could take several months to disappear. The compression garments have to work for a longer time as well, because we don't want to increase the possibility that blood clots could occur. These garments are very tight and can be very difficult to get on, but even though they are frustrating, it's essential that they are worn.

Q: *Do all liposuction doctors perform this surgery?*

A: No. It is somewhat more complicated and risky to work on calves and ankles. It's extremely important to make sure your surgeon has had experience in these areas, because this surgery is not suited for beginning surgeons or surgeons who have never done calves and ankles before.

Q: *How long do patients have to be in the office for these procedures?*

A: It's hard to estimate, because you are working in a tight area. A good estimate would be two to three hours, but it could be more, depending on the specific patient and how slowly the surgeon has to work.

POINTS TO REMEMBER

• Always ask your surgeon about his or her experience doing liposuction on the part of the body you want done. Not all surgeons are experienced in every area.

- Liposuction is performed on many different areas of the body, and each procedure is slightly different.

- The facial jowls and neck can be noticeably improved when excess fat is present, although some people might need a face-lift as well.

- Liposuction on the arms, especially on the backs of the upper arms, is often performed in women, especially those in their late 40s and older.

- Liposuction is often used for breast reduction in men. In women, the procedure can be risky, and those contemplating it should be very cautious.

- Many women have liposuction on the upper back, especially those over 50, and feel more comfortable in clothing afterward.

- People with excess fat on their flanks, the sides of the trunk, can benefit from liposuction.

- The waist and hips can be done with the flanks to create a smooth, curved contour.

- Removal of excess fat in the belly is a common procedure. Sometimes a tummy tuck is also needed, but it should be done at a separate time.

- Working on the buttocks is challenging because of different concepts of what an aesthetic buttock's proportions should be, and surgeons try to achieve the shape the patient desires. Significant fat removal is possible in this area, but not in the thigh right under the buttock, for fear that the buttock will droop.

- Thighs are also commonly done, especially the "saddle-bags" on the outer thighs.

- Knees, calves, and ankles can also benefit from liposuction, although these areas might have more swelling and take longer to heal.

12

• WHAT HAPPENS AFTER LIPOSUCTION

AS you have been reading this book, you have learned about some of the things you need to do following your liposuction procedure. In this chapter, we will review the instructions that have been discussed and let you know about other things you should and should not do.

Q: *How long do you need to have someone with you after the procedure?*

A: You should have someone with you for the first 24 hours. During that time, you should never be left alone. You should make arrangements to have someone take you home, even if you use a car service or taxi. The person staying at home with you should remain at least until you have taken your first shower and dressed, and not leave you alone until 24 hours after the procedure.

Q: *What should you do in that first 24 hours?*

A: The best thing to do is stay home and rest. You need to relax on the evening and the day after liposuction. However, you should not spend all your time in bed. You need to get up and walk around for at least a few minutes every hour, except when you go to sleep. This bit of activity fosters the healing process by helping more anesthetic fluid to drain out, which contributes to less bruising and increases your circulation, lessening the already low risk of developing blood clots.

Q: *When can you resume normal activity?*

A: Most people can move around normally after two days.

Q: *How long does drainage from the insertion sites last?*

A: It's different with everyone, but it is normal to have some fluids draining out during the first one or two days, especially while you are walking around your house.

Q: *Is there anything special you should do if you had liposuction on your extremities?*

A: If your arms, knees, or lower legs were treated, you must keep them elevated for the first 12 hours after surgery whenever you are not moving around. When you are at rest, your arms, knees, or lower legs have to be higher than your heart. You should do this at all times, except for the brief times when you are taking your walks, using the bathroom, or eating.

Q: *Is it common to have pain or discomfort?*

A: You will probably feel sore for several days after liposuction, but as you wear the compression garment, you will find the discomfort lessens. If you are bothered, you can take Tylenol if your doctor has approved it.

Some people also have what we call "hot spots," which are small areas near the treated sites that are sore. Ice can be used (10 minutes on, 20 minutes off) for the first few days. Thereafter, warm compresses might help lessen the discomfort. You can gently massage these spots (other than the neck) beginning five days after the procedure. In other cases, you can go to the doctor's office for a warm external ultrasound treatment.

If you have any severe pain, which is quite rare, you should let your doctor know immediately.

Q: *What should you do if you have continuing pain, a fever, or other symptoms you don't expect?*

A: If anything happens that concerns you or that you think is unusual, you should call the doctor's office right away. It's extremely rare for patients to experience any serious side effects on the first day after liposuction. Even so, if you observe anything unusual, you should contact your doctor immediately and describe what is going on to be certain that nothing is wrong.

Q: *Will everyone have bruising and swelling?*

A: Both are completely normal. Bruising might not appear for a few days, and swelling around the areas treated is always expected. Bruising and swelling can also occur in areas other than those treated. With liposuction on the lower belly, bruising and swelling can occur on the labia, penis, and scrotum; with lower legs, on the feet; and with upper arms, on the forearms. An athletic supporter can help men who have swelling in the scrotum.

Q: *Is it common to feel dizzy during that first 24 hours after surgery?*

A: You might feel dizzy if you stand up too quickly or move in a sudden or jerky manner. For that reason, you should always get up very slowly from a chair, the bed, or the toilet and make sure that someone is standing right by you during that first 24 hours. This is especially a concern when you first remove the compression garment and take your first shower (see below).

Q: *Is there anything special you have to know about your diet after surgery?*

A: During the first 24 hours, you must drink at least a quart of water. During that same time period, you should also carefully avoid any beverages that have caffeine, including coffee, tea, and soda.

For the first two weeks, you should also limit foods that are high in salt, such as Chinese food and pizza, because salt is involved in liquid retention and can prolong the healing period.

Q: *What if you're a smoker?*

A: You should not smoke cigarettes, cigars, or pipes for at least one week after the procedure. You should also avoid secondhand smoke, because the smoke deprives your blood of oxygen, which could result in scarring.

Q: *Do you have to take any medication?*

A: Yes, you have to continue to take the antibiotics that were prescribed until you have finished taking the full prescription. If you were taking any medications that you did not have to stop for the procedure, you should just continue taking them. Most medications that were stopped for a week prior to the procedure can be resumed one week after the procedure, and those that were stopped two days before can be resumed two days after. Check with your doctor to be certain.

Q: *Do you need any extra vitamins while you're healing?*

A: If you don't already take one, you should take a multivitamin every day for four weeks after the procedure. That will promote good healing.

Q: *How long do you have to wear your compression garment?*

A: In most cases, the garment should be worn 24 hours a day, seven days a week for two weeks. Then, during weeks three and four, it should be worn for 12 hours a day, either in the day or the night. Neck garments must be worn for 24 hours for the first two days at least. Then they must be worn at night for two weeks. Many patients feel better and may develop a better result by wearing the garment for six weeks.

Q: *What happens if you don't wear the garment or wear it only part of the time recommended?*

A: If your compression garment is not worn for the prescribed number of hours and length of time, your swelling will get worse and it will take you longer to heal. At times these garments can be uncomfortable or difficult to put on or take off, but the results are well worth the trouble. You should have someone assist you with them, if possible, and you should always remove them slowly after you have eaten.

Q: *How do you take care of your insertion sites?*

A: At the office, we leave them open, putting dressing on them to absorb the leaking fluid. It is your responsibility to keep your wounds covered with dressing at all times. That means you have to place a large, absorbent dressing over all your incision sites for about three or four days after surgery, until they are no longer leaking fluid.

You also have to keep the wounds moist by putting a prescribed antibiotic ointment on them. The morning after your procedure, you remove the dressing the office has placed on and then you have to change the dressing twice a day until the sites are completely healed. Exact instructions for doing this are provided by the doctor's office.

If the insertion sites are sutured, they will be covered by sterile tape, and you can leave these strips alone. In that case, a drainage insertion may be created at the lowest point of the surgery, and this is left open and treated as mentioned in the paragraph above.

Q: *When can you take a shower or bath?*

A: You may take a shower the morning after your procedure. At that time, you should slowly remove your compression garment, remain seated for five minutes, then stand up gradually. Remember that someone must be with you at this time to make sure you don't fall and hurt yourself. Consider using a folding chair in the shower for added safety. If you feel faint, sit down until you feel all right again. After your shower, dry off, dress the insertion sites with ointment and Band-Aids, and put on a clean compression garment. You should not take a bath or sit in a hot tub or whirlpool until all your insertion sites are healed (several days to two weeks or more).

Q: *When can you go back to your exercise routine?*

A: On the first day after surgery, you can do light exercise, such as limited walking. You should not bend, strain, pull, push, or lift heavy items for a week after surgery. You can go back to a gradual exercise program, with the exception of swimming, a few days after the procedure. Vigorous exercise should not be attempted for one week after surgery.

You should never strain yourself. Be aware of your body, and stop immediately if you feel any pain or unusual discomfort. Avoid that particular exercise and then try it again in a few days. Of course, you will also be wearing your compression garments while you exercise.

Q: *What if you swim?*

A: You must not swim while your insertion sites are healing—not in a pool, pond, lake, ocean, or anywhere else. Otherwise, you might develop an infection, which could be hard to treat. Most people can go back to swimming 7 to 14 days after their procedure, unless the insertion sites are not fully healed. Your doctor will let you know.

Q: *When can you resume sexual relations?*

A: You should not have sex until after all your insertion sites have healed. If birth control pills were discontinued prior to surgery, resume them at the next appropriate cycle and use an additional form of birth control for the first cycle. You should also consult your gynecologist about how to proceed.

Q: *Does everyone have some scarring?*

A: Yes, because liposuction involves insertions into the skin. Anytime you do that, the skin will scar. A lot of it depends on how well the individual patient heals. Most heal with a small, hard-to-see fine line. Even if tiny scars develop, as thick or darker-colored scars, they may be hidden in creases or folds of the skin or they may be in areas that are not normally visible or covered by clothing.

Sometimes, these scars can become red or raised or after a year or two and get darker in color. There are various techniques that can improve their appearance, such as dressings, creams, laser and excisional scar revision, so if you have any scarring that troubles you, discuss it with your surgeon.

Q: *What is the biggest postsurgical mistake people make?*

A: Thinking of liposuction as a weight reduction method and not following a healthy diet and regular exercise program afterward. Most people will be extra careful about this, in view of the time, effort, and expense they have devoted to improving their appearance with this surgery. Those who choose to ignore their diet and exercise and gain weight afterward are definitely making a mistake.

POINTS TO REMEMBER

- Someone should be with you at all times for the first 24 hours following surgery.

- Arms, knees, and lower legs that have undergone liposuction must be elevated for the first 12 hours after surgery.

- You might have soreness or some discomfort for a few days, but pain is not normally experienced.

- If you have any unusual or unexpected side effects, notify your doctor's office immediately.

- Almost everyone has some degree of bruising and swelling.

- After surgery, you should have no caffeine for two days, should not eat salty foods for one week, and should not smoke for one week. A daily multivitamin for the first four weeks is also recommended.

- Compression garments must be worn for several weeks to allow your body to heal properly.

- Insertion sites must be treated with ointment and kept covered for a few days until they heal.

- You can resume most exercise programs in a week, but you must be careful to avoid strain.

- Most people have some scars at their insertion sites. Treatment to improve them is available when needed.

- People who mistakenly think that liposuction is for weight loss might ignore diet and exercise afterward and gain back fat. Enlightened patients know better!

- Always follow your doctor's postsurgical instructions to the letter if you want to achieve the best results and remain healthy.

13

• POSSIBLE SIDE EFFECTS AND COMPLICATIONS

AS we have told you, tumescent liposuction is a remarkably safe procedure. A recent national survey of 66,570 liposuction procedures found no deaths and serious adverse effects in only 0.68 per 1,000 cases—less than 1 percent. This survey, published in *Dermatologic Surgery*, the journal of the American Society for Dermatologic Surgery, concluded that "office-based tumescent liposuction performed by dermatologic surgeons is safe, with a lower complication rate than hospital-based procedures."

But that doesn't mean liposuction surgery is a piece of cake. Just about everyone will experience some side effects, normal responses to surgery that go away as the body heals. In rare cases, however, medical complications can develop. In this chapter, we will discuss the side effects you can expect and the complications that can occur when things don't go quite right.

Q: *What should people know about possible side effects or complications that can occur with liposuction?*

A: There is every possibility that you will be very happy with your surgery and its results, and you will get back to your regular activities quickly. But that might take longer for some people than for others. There can be persistent soreness in certain areas, irregularities in skin tone, a subtle indentation here or there, or darker pigmentation at the insertion sites. There is usually some bruising and swelling; drainage from insertion sites can last for up to 24 hours.

You might also be happy with one side of your body and not happy with the other side. In other words, things might not look entirely symmetrical, or the skin might appear smoother or the contour more pleasing on one side than on the other. Or maybe you think not enough fat was removed.

There are also some complications that can occur from time to time, and it's a good thing for patients to know about them in advance. They can include seromas, which are collections of fluid underneath the skin. Infections are very rare, but they have occurred in a few cases. Patients need to understand that liposuction is surgery and with any surgery, even the safest, unwanted side effects and complications occasionally happen. There are no guarantees. Everyone heals differently. Even the same patient might heal differently when liposuction is done on different areas.

Q: *Can you briefly define the difference between side effects and complications?*

A: Side effects are anticipated things that happen as a result of the procedure. They might not happen in all patients, but if they do happen, they are expected and are not a true complication.

Complications are more serious conditions that happen uncommonly as a result of surgery. There can be many different causes, including undiagnosed medical problems, anatomical irregularities, infections, bleeding, failure to follow postsurgical instructions, and physician errors.

Side Effects

Q: *What are some of the more common side effects patients can expect following their surgery?*

A: First of all, we should warn people not to become worried or overly concerned when they hear about possible side effects, because either they are minor and soon disappear, or in some cases, they don't happen at all. We have to discuss all of them in case they happen, so patients can be prepared.

We have already mentioned quite a few, including bruising, swelling, tenderness, numbness, or increased sensitivity that could become permanent in some areas, skin dimpling, cellulite appearing more obvious, dents, depressions, lumpiness, hardness, small scars at the insertion sites that might darken with sun exposure or become tender or itchy, slight asymmetry, bleeding, hematomas (collections of blood under the skin which require draining), friction blisters from dressings, seromas (accumulations of serum that require draining), dizziness and fainting, fatigue and depressions, slight temperature increase during first 48 hours, and flushing of the face.

Q: *Most people worry about pain. Does it occur after liposuction?*

A: Pain can occur, but it's very variable, with most people having minimal discomfort, other having a sore area for which they may take an over-the-counter anti-inflammatory medication. That can last for a few days to a few weeks. But most patients do not complain of "pain."

Q: *How long do patients have swelling?*

A: The fluid swelling goes down in the first few days, and as it's going down, the surgical swelling is increasing, so you might not see a difference. In fact, you might not observe a diminution of the swelling for a few weeks. The biggest reduction might be in the first 12 hours. Then, over the next several weeks, you will observe the swelling gradually going down.

Q: *How long does bruising and tenderness last?*

A: All surgical patients have some tenderness to the touch for a short term in the surgical area. Like bruising, it might last for a day or two. The bruising might show up immediately, or it might not be evident until one to three days after the procedure. This bruising, as we have mentioned, can also be in areas other than those we worked on. Liposuction right under the neck, for example, can result in bruising on the lower part of the neck going down to the collarbone. Bruising does not cause any permanent problems and clears on its own. On the face, it might take a week and a half to disappear, and on the lower body, it can take up to three weeks. The color of the bruising goes through normal stages of changing color from very purple to green and yellow and then clearing.

Q: *Does everyone have oozing of fluids after the procedure?*

A: Yes. Right after surgery, when patients first stand up to be checked, the fluid, which consists mostly of anesthetic and a very few red blood cells, does come out. Because it has a few blood cells, it's usually pink, but sometimes it looks red. Patients need to know that the fluid is not their blood coming out. This drainage can continue for about 24 hours, but for some people it is a much shorter time.

Q: *What kinds of scars appear on the insertion sites?*

A: All insertion sites leave tiny scars. It's impossible to do surgery by making an opening in the skin without creating a scar. In many cases, these scars are tiny and almost impossible to see, but in some people, or in certain parts of the body, they might heal with a white scar, a dark scar, or a scar that becomes raised several months later. Remember that when we select the insertion sites, we try to find spots that will be hidden, so for most people, these small scars are not a problem. Just about everyone has some scars. Maybe they burned themselves with an iron or hot pot in the kitchen; maybe they accidentally nicked themselves with a razor or cut their finger with a knife. People have these small scars for years and don't even notice them.

Q: Why do some scars get dark?

A: They pigment. They become not just red, which is normal for a short time, but they turn darker brown. It's the body reacting to the trauma of injury to the skin, which is what happens with any surgery. If these dark scars are visible and bother the patient, they can be treated and improved later on.

Q: How long do patients have tenderness and numbness?

A: Typically, they resolve over several months or sometimes longer. In very rare cases, there might be patches of skin that retain numbness permanently, but that won't interfere with function.

Q: Can you explain friction blisters?

A: They often occur from wearing the compression garment too tightly. That can cause creases in the skin, which could become long-term indentations, as the garment digs into the skin and forms grooves. So if there is too much tension, the garment can produce blisters. They don't cause long-term problems by themselves, but they should be treated with antibiotic ointment.

Q: *How does liposuction affect skin irregularities?*

A: If they were pre-existing, like cellulite, it's possible that they might become worse after the procedure, but generally, they remain unchanged and rarely improve. Remember that liposuction is not a treatment to improve these irregularities. On occasion, liposuction can also cause them, including indentations, dimpling, dents, and depressions.

Q: *You also mentioned lumpiness and hardness of the skin.*

A: They can occur in patchy areas after surgery because of inflammation. The inflammation creates swelling, and when there is swelling under the tissues, it creates a hardness when you feel your skin from above. In most cases, it goes away after a few months. In extremely rare cases, fibrosis, or scarring, occurs deeply and remains as a hard lump. This might be due to the patient's overhealing tendency.

Q: *What about itching?*

A: Some patients definitely have itching in the first few days after surgery. It might be a result of the healing, the compression garment they have to wear, or the disinfectant that is used on their skin. This can be treated with an antihistamine.

Q: *How frequent is dizziness and fainting?*

A: Sometimes, during the first 24 hours after surgery, patients might feel dizzy or even faint. It often happens the next day when they take off their garments to bathe. The garment has been applying pressure, which squeezes on the blood vessels within the fat area. When they remove the garment, the blood vessels begin to engorge and more blood goes to that area and less to the head. That's why patients should never be alone for the first 24 hours. There is no guarantee that they might not feel lightheaded if they quickly remove their garment and then step into the shower. You certainly don't want to fall down on a hard tile surface.

Fainting is far less common, but it has happened. That's why you should sit down, remove the garment very slowly, and remain seated for a few minutes before you stand up. Then stand up slowly, make sure you are steady, and move your legs a little to keep the blood flowing for a minute before you get into the shower. As we previously suggested, using a chair in the shower can be an added safety factor. Make sure you don't feel dizzy and that you are stable before you stand, walk, and shower.

Q: *Are fatigue and depression common side effects?*

A: Anyone going through surgery has a normal amount of their own adrenaline flowing during the procedure; it's the "fight or flight" phenomenon as your adrenal glands produce adrenaline to give you added energy to deal with the upcoming event. Once the procedure is over, the adrenaline level decreases and you might experience a "letdown" as it returns to its normal level. As a result, you might feel sluggish and tired.

Other people might feel depressed as well, asking themselves, *Why did I do this to myself? I'm swollen, I'm bruised, I'm leaking, I'm sore. Why did I do it?* Many patients feel this way for a day or two, if it happens. It doesn't usually last longer than that. It's not as common with liposuction as it is with procedures like face-lifts, but people should be aware of it in case they start to experience these feelings.

Q: *You mentioned an elevated temperature or flushing.*

A: On the evening of surgery, some people have a flushing or redness in their face and upper neck. It goes away by the next day. Others have a slightly elevated temperature for the first 48 hours; this is not a fever, but a very mild and temporary change by one degree or so. Others have a very slight elevation in their pulse and heart rates, neither of which is life-threatening, just a normal and temporary side effect for some.

Q: *Do some women have menstrual irregularities?*

A: Many women find that their cycle can be thrown off a little bit in the first month or two after surgery. It goes back on schedule again.

Complications

Q: *Are side effects and complications related?*

A: In some cases, yes. Side effects that do not go away with time, that remain or get worse, can become complications.

Q: *Do these include skin irregularities?*

A: They can. Aside from minimal irregularities, there can be significant depressions because of the way the patient was lying or positioned during surgery, or if their underling bony framework was pushing the fat up too high. So even though the correct amount of fat was apparently removed during surgery, once the patient stands, it becomes evident that there is now a depression in their contour.

The size of these depressions can be small, like the indentation of the finger or as large as the size of the palm. The good news is that these depressions can be improved with fat injections (see chapter nineteen).

Q: *Please explain how seromas form.*

A: Seromas occur when a collection of fluid forms underneath the skin. This fluid consists of serum or blood and forms bumps that are felt but might not be seen. Seromas, which are masses formed by the collection of fluid in the tissues usually at the site of a wound, can be soft or firm, depending on how much fluid they contain. A seroma might go away on its own, but it often needs to be drained a series of times with a very fine needle. Then a dressing is put on for compression, and the patient comes back until there is no further accumulation of fluid. It's possible that some people are more prone to develop seromas than others. They are not common with tumescent liposuction, but they do occur more often with internal ultrasonic-assisted liposuction.

Q: *What about hematomas?*

A: Hematomas are masses of clotted blood that can occur with bleeding under the skin. They occur very rarely with liposuction and excisional surgery. When people have surgery, there's normal oozing of red blood cells through the insertion sites, and some of those cells can accumulate and cause a bruising discoloration. But if a blood vessel is disturbed, a greater amount of blood could collect and harden into a clot, forming a hematoma.

Warm compresses might be sufficient treatment, but sometimes the hematoma can cause problems and might have to be removed through a small incision and a needle.

With tumescent liposuction techniques, however, hematomas rarely occur unless the patient is overly active during the first 24 hours, which could cause one to form.

Q: *You said that in some cases, permanent numbness can occur.*

A: It is possible that even a few years after liposuction, some people might have an area of permanent numbness. It doesn't affect muscular function, but if you scratch the skin in that area, you might not feel it.

Q: *Can liposuction ever affect nerve function?*

A: There is a rare complication when liposuction is performed on the neck. The surgery can cause a nerve impairment, so that when a person smiles, their mouth opens, but on the side of the surgery that affected the nerve, part of the lower lip will not come down with the smile. Very often when this happens, it is only a temporary condition. It's like the nerve has gone into hibernation because it has experienced trauma in its neighborhood. The nerve itself hasn't been injured, however, and in a few days to a few weeks or even months, its activity will increase and once again be normal. This condition is very rarely permanent.

Q: *You mentioned darkening of scars. Are there ever permanent pigmentation changes in the skin following liposuction?*

A: Pigmentation, or darkening of the insertion sites, can occasionally occur, especially in those individuals with naturally darker skin, those with brown eyes, and those patients who get a sunburns. This usually resolves itself within several months, but it can take more than a year. I have seen permanent pigmentation in people who have been burned by irons, especially on the lower body. It is possible for someone to develop a permanent brown scar on an insertion site. There is treatment to deal with this problem should it occur.

Q: *Can serious infections ever occur?*

A: Infections happen less than 1 percent of the time. Most physicians prescribe antibiotics around the time of surgery. The tumescent anesthetic also has antibacterial properties. But if an infection does occur, it can be for several different reasons. Perhaps the patient's immune system isn't strong. Or they might have undiagnosed diabetes or fail to take care of their wounds carefully. Some people have liposuction by nonlicensed providers, and the equipment might not be properly sterilized. Patients might also have an underlying medical condition of which they are not aware.

Once again, you have to recognize the fact that life-threatening infections can occur with every kind of surgery that exists—even liposuction—but they are extremely rare—less than 1 percent. These infections can be treated with antibiotics and possible draining. No surgeon can guarantee that it is impossible for you to develop an infection. It's just very unlikely.

Q: *What about another serious complication, pulmonary emboli?*

A: When fat particles travel to the lung, they are called pulmonary emboli. They are exceedingly rare, but they have occurred when tumescent liposuction is performed with another procedure such as a tummy tuck, especially if the patient is under general anesthesia, is immobile and not moving during the surgery, and is also on the birth control pill and smokes. When you combine all these risk factors, especially if they also have a family history of something similar, pulmonary emboli can occur. This is a life-threatening condition.

A similar situation with blood clots in the legs can cause serious problems, but if patients are awake and moving, as they are during tumescent liposuction, this complication should not happen.

Q: *Can liposuction ever have dangerous effects on the heart?*

A: It is possible that a patient could have an underlying heart rhythm disorder that is triggered by the adrenaline in the anesthetic. If a patient develops toxicity at a high level of the anesthetic, perhaps because they were taking another medication and the physician was not aware of it, it is possible that the high level of anesthetic could create problems with the heart and the patient's ability to breathe. But again, this has been well studied and is extremely rare with tumescent liposuction.

Q: *Are patients ever allergic to anything used in the liposuction procedure?*

A: There is an extremely rare possibility that a patient could have an allergic reaction to the medications that are given, such as the antibiotic. They could develop hives, respiratory distress, or shortness of breath. It is extremely rare that anyone has an allergic reaction to lidocaine, but it is possible that if they have a sulfa allergy, they might be allergic to the preservative in the anesthetic, and a referral to an allergist for testing may be necessary. That's why it is so vital that patients tell their doctors about any and all allergies they have. In a case like this, the doctor would be able to use an alternative anesthetic that does not contain that preservative.

Q: *Can you summarize what you think potential patients should try to remember about side effects and complications from liposuction?*

A: Tumescent liposuction is an extremely safe procedure. The common side effects we've discussed are generally short in duration, and the complications are very rare.

Given that, it is extremely important that if patients have any concerns, if things do not seem to be going according to schedule, or if they have even the slightest concern about anything, they should not hesitate to call the doctor's office immediately. Excellent communication is vital to the team effort of physician, staff, and patient and leads to the best end results.

POINTS TO REMEMBER

- There are many possible side effects from liposuction, and they can last from a few hours to a few months or more.

- Rare complications can occur at times, as with any surgical procedure.

- Patients should be well informed in advance about possible side effects and complications.

- Actual pain is very rare. Minor discomfort is more common and can last from a few days to a few weeks.

- Common side effects include bruising, swelling, and drainage of fluids.

- Everyone gets some degree of scarring at the insertions sites, but it is often not easily seen. Problem areas can be treated and improved.

- Other possible side effects include skin tenderness, numbness, lumpiness, hardness, itching, fatigue, dizziness, fainting, depression, flushing, slightly elevated temperature, and menstrual irregularities.

- Side effects that do not resolve with time can turn into complications.

- Seromas, collections of fluid under the skin, can resolve on their own or might require draining.

- Hematomas, masses of clotted blood under the skin, are rare with liposuction and might require draining.

- A small number of patients can develop permanent numbness in one area.

- Infections from liposuction are very rare and occur less than 1 percent of the time.

- Extremely rarely, patients might be allergic to the medications or anesthetic used for liposuction.

- It is vital that patients immediately contact their doctor's office if anything—even something that seems minor—concerns them.

14

• HOW TO EVALUATE YOUR RESULTS

IN earlier chapters, we talked about the importance of realistic expectations. Liposuction is not a miracle procedure and might not be able to create the exact body you dream about. But it can make a big difference by removing stubborn areas of fat that you can't get off with diet and exercise. You will lose weight—although not a great deal—and you will lose inches. You may even drop a dress size. If you are like most people, you will definitely look better. Liposuction can make a big difference, and people will notice.

But how do you evaluate your results? How should you look right after the procedure? A week later? A few weeks later, after your body is healing and the swelling has gone down? Did the procedure work properly? Did all the excess fat come out? Are there any remaining areas that concern you? After your procedure, you will want to ask yourself these and many other questions. In this chapter, we will guide you in evaluating your results.

Q: *How long should patients wait before trying to assess liposuction results?*

A: To some extent, you will see and feel immediate improvement. During the procedure, you can see your fat coming out and going into a bottle. You can't remove fat and be the same afterward. Something has to improve. So even though patients are somewhat swollen from the anesthetic, they can usually tell by looking at themselves and by feeling the fat between their fingers that they have definitely lost unwanted fat.

Q: *Can patients evaluate their results during the first few weeks?*

A: During that time, the swelling from the surgery will increase, especially if they don't wear a compression garment. If they do wear the garment, the skin will retract further and pull closer to the muscle, becoming denser and tighter. This process goes on for three to six months. After six months, there is seldom any additional improvement, so at that point, you can make a full assessment of your results.

Q: *How much should patients improve?*

A: That varies from patient to patient and also from body site to body site. Some peoples' appearance might look less dramatic when they take fat out of one area, such as the outer thigh. The contour might change, and the patient might be very happy, but it might not be that noticeable to others. Weight loss also varies. Some people see no change in their weight on the scale but feel as though they have lost five pounds. There are even some people who go down two sizes in clothing. So there is quite a wide variation in the results people can get from liposuction.

Q: *Then how can people assess their results?*

A: The first thing to look at is the improvement in how you feel in clothing. In the area or areas that bothered you, do your clothes now fit better? When you look in the mirror, is your contour more pleasing? Some liposuction patients have to buy whole new wardrobes or have all their clothes taken in. For some people, the result is a dramatic improvement. For others, it might be more subtle.

The best way to assess your results is not by looking down at yourself while standing, but by looking straight ahead at yourself as you stand in front of a full-length mirror. After all, that's the way other people see you. When you look down at your body, you see different curves, whereas people generally look at you while you are in an upright position.

Q: *What are some of the factors that can affect the quality of your results?*

A: There are a few physical characteristics that can limit your ability to get superior results, including large bony framework, cellulite, large muscle mass, loose skin, severe stretch marks, scoliosis or curvature of the spine, and contour waviness due to irregular fatty deposits.

Q: *How should you evaluate your body in the first two weeks?*

A: Look for equalness from side to side. Look for evenness of the curvature. Do you see any significant depressions? How are your insertion scars healing? Are any of them still open? Look at the coloration in your skin. If there was bruising, is it going away? Can you find any lumpiness? Hardness? In general, how is the quality of your skin?

A big part of the assessment is asking yourself if you are happy with your new body. Does it look that way you want it to? Does the area where you had liposuction blend into the adjacent areas of your body? Or is something wrong with the proportion? Do other parts of your body that were not worked on now look out of proportion? Do you think they might also need work?

Make a note of everything you see, the things you like and the things that bother you, and bring them to your surgeon when you go back for a follow-up examination.

Q: *Does the surgeon automatically look at all these things when you return for your follow-up visit?*

A: The first visit after liposuction is usually between a week and two weeks later. At that time, we are assessing mainly medical factors. Is there any evidence of infection? Are there any seromas or hematomas? Is the bruising normal and improving? Are the insertion scars healing properly? Is the compression garment being worn properly? Is there any tenderness or soreness when you work out? Is there any lumpiness that might require special treatment (see chapter fifteen). We also ask the patient if there is anything unusual that should be brought to our attention.

Q: *What do doctors look for at the next visit?*

A: Depending on how patients are healing, the next visit may not be until three months after the procedure. At that point, we are definitely looking at the shape or contour of the body in the area where we worked. We look at the skin elasticity and see if it is redraping into a somewhat tight position. We look to see if there is still any sagging skin or if it has retracted.

Is there any additional fat we did not or could not remove during the first procedure? Does this patient need a secondary liposuction procedure? We are also looking for medical things, such as localized swelling, lumpiness, or any of the other possible side effects we discussed.

Q: *If someone needs a secondary procedure, when would it be done?*

A: I don't usually perform them until at least six months after the first procedure. Patients need time to heal completely and also to evaluate their treatment, decide if there is more to be done, and reduce that area to its minimal amount. You should know that studies indicate that there is a 10 to 12 percent chance that liposuction patients may need a secondary procedure.

Q: *If you follow a good diet and exercise program, is it still possible that the fat could come back to the same areas where you had it removed?*

A: It is possible, but it often does not happen that way. When liposuction is done, significant amounts of fat cells are removed but, by design, not all of them. We need fat for circulation, insulation, and to protect the overlying skin. The fat cells that remain are alive and can certainly store more fat if the patient consumes enough calories. But that doesn't mean all the fat that patients might regain goes to the area where liposuction was done.

More often, added fat is generally deposited in areas such as the upper body, legs, or tummy, depending on where the patient had surgery. In other words, some of the fat will go to the area where it was removed, but it will be distributed to other areas as well, instead of concentrating on one or two areas. As an example, some women, especially after abdominal liposuction, find that their breasts enlarge, sometimes even without any change in diet or weight gain. But that doesn't happen for every woman, and the reasons why it happens for some are not clear.

Q: *What causes people to gain weight after liposuction?*

A: People who have put on weight after liposuction have to make sure they haven't relied on liposuction as a substitute for diet and exercise and that they continue to exercise and eat a healthy diet. If they consume more calories than they did before surgery, they will put on weight, and it can go to the area where they had the procedure as well as other areas of the body.

Another thing to remember is that after liposuction, depending on how much fat you had removed, you don't need the same number of calories per day to maintain your weight—you need less. So if you go back to eating exactly what you ate before—especially if you had a relatively large amount of fat removed—you will probably gain weight if your exercise program remains the same. You should be aware that one study showed that although more than a third of liposuction patients maintained their weight loss after the procedure, a little less than half gained back some weight. You really have to be diligent.

Q: *Do you perform liposuction again in the same areas when people regain the fat?*

A: It is possible, but it's also important for a patient to demonstrate their willingness to be committed to a lifelong regimen of eating healthy and exercising. Yo-yo dieting—losing and gaining weight over and over again—is very dangerous for your health.

POINTS TO REMEMBER

- You can see and feel improvement immediately after surgery.

- Swelling during the first weeks might make it difficult to assess your final results.

- After six months, there is usually no further improvement, so you can fully evaluate your results.

- Improvement varies from person to person and from one body area to another.

- Some people see weight loss, while others see only contour changes. Some go down one or even two sizes in clothing and need a new wardrobe.

- The way your clothing fits and feels are important measures of liposuction's success.

- Patients and surgeons should assess a list of different medical and aesthetic factors in the weeks and months following liposuction.

• Sometimes a secondary procedure is recommended to remove additional fat deposits.

• Weight gained after liposuction might return to the area that was worked on, but it is usually more generally distributed to several areas of the body.

15

• WHAT CAN BE DONE IF YOU'RE UNHAPPY WITH YOUR RESULTS

A good surgeon will make every effort to see that you are happy with the results of your liposuction procedure. Sometimes, a secondary procedure will be performed to correct problems. In other cases, a different form of treatment might be used to make improvements. It's important that you know what options are available if you want or need to have more work done. In this chapter, we will talk about some of the things patients might want to change after liposuction, whether they can be changed, and if so, how that can be accomplished.

Q: *What are some legitimate complaints that liposuction patients might have?*

A: There are some body areas where there is stubborn, resistant fat that seems to persist, for example, around the belly button, the nipple, the rolls of fat on the upper back, and also male breasts and love handles. There is fibrous skin in these areas, and at times they cannot be improved past a certain point. So sometimes patients want more reduced, but it might not be possible. In some cases, the liposuction procedure did not remove all the excess fat, so we will go in a second time to get it out.

In addition, there might be areas with a notch or indentation that can be improved with fat injections or other small procedures (see chapter nineteen).

Q: *What if someone insists that more fat can be removed when that is not the case?*

A: They might simply need more explanation and education. Or they might have a psychological disorder, such as body dysmorphic tendency, where they believe they are fat when in fact, they are not.

Q: *What do you say to patients who are unhappy because they think not enough fat was removed?*

A: I can only respond with the facts. As a surgeon, I do the absolute best I can for each patient and remove as much fat as I think can be removed *safely*. I will not put my patients at risk for complications because they want to use liposuction to take off a lot of excess weight—weight they can take off themselves with diet and exercise.

So if someone isn't happy with the amount of fat that has been removed, I examine that patient and see if I agree.

If I do, we can schedule a secondary procedure. If I don't, I'll explain exactly why to the patient. Also, remember that most often, these matters are discussed prior to liposuction and patients have a pretty clear picture of how much fat they can expect to lose and what kind of contour they will achieve.

Q: *What do you have to find out about why patients are unhappy?*

A: We have to discover if the reason for their dissatisfaction is because not enough fat was removed. If that is the case and more can be removed, then we can do that. But if we took out as much as we could and the patients are still not happy, we have to go back and talk about expectations again and try to re-educate them regarding what can and cannot be done safely. Patients have to be reassured that we have done everything we can do in that area, if that is the case.

There are also patients who are unhappy because they think too much fat was removed. The area might be depressed or out of balance with surrounding areas. If that is the case, we can often improve it with fat injections (see chapter nineteen) or smooth it out by removing a little more fat in the right spots.

Q: *What are some important facts that unhappy patients should know?*

A: Do not immediately run to another physician if you have any problems after liposuction. The first thing to do is continue to communicate with the surgeon who did your procedure. Things do happen after surgery and everyone heals differently, so people should make a point of addressing all their concerns with their doctor and trying to work it out before they do anything else. After all, no other doctor can possibly know as much as your surgeon about how your procedure was done.

Second, some of their complaints may not be sound or realistic. They might think they have some additional fat, but it might actually be muscle or bone and the contour can't be changed any further. Or they might have complaints about things that are only temporary and they just need to be reassured that over time, these things will improve or go away entirely. Patients often need to be patient!

You should also be aware that some unhappiness is a result of seeing disproportion in the area that has been worked on once that spot is reduced. In other words, the liposuction was successful, but now other areas seem too big. For example, maybe your hips didn't bother you before surgery, but now that your outer thighs have been done and are smaller, you are suddenly bothered by the size of your hips. So you are happy with your thighs, but unhappy because now your hips appear to be projecting out much farther. If that is the case, you might want to have a procedure on your hips in the future.

And finally, there are people who are unhappy because of coincidences.

Q: *What kinds of coincidences?*

A: Let's say someone has liposuction and a few days later, breaks out with shingles or hives. There is no connection with the surgery, but the patient thinks there is. That's when communication with your physician is so important. Always let your doctor know about *all* your concerns, explain what's bothering you, no matter how small it might be, and give the doctor a chance to examine you and offer an evaluation. Whatever is troubling you might not be what you think it is, and it might have no connection to your procedure.

Q: *Is there any way for patients to get a clearer picture of how things will look after additional procedures?*

A: Some surgeons are adept at using computer imaging. They take pictures of their patients, put them on the screen, and modify the pictures to present an idea of how they will look. But this procedure can backfire, because as we know, liposuction does not always come out exactly the way we expect or want it to. So I don't use this procedure because I don't want to give my patients false hopes or expectations. We know areas of fat will come down, and we can give them an average, but that might not be precisely what happens for them.

Q: *If there is more fat to remove, what happens?*

A: It is important to wait a minimum of six months after the first procedure so the body can heal to the maximum possible extent. Sometimes we even wait for a year. Then we can go back and do more.

Q: *What is that second procedure like for the patient?*

A: Sometimes it can be more uncomfortable. The fat in the area where we worked might have become more fibrous, and adhesions and scar tissue can form within the fatty layer. So it might be a little more difficult to numb the area, and patients can feel an occasional twinge here or there during the procedure. Of course, we can always put more anesthetic in when that happens.

Q: *Is a secondary procedure the same thing as a revision or touch-up?*

A: Yes. There are also times when a person has surgery that is planned in stages, so a secondary procedure is expected. A touch-up could be done in a small area where there might be an excess lump we want to take out, but we don't use that term because it sounds as though what we're going to do will only take a minute.

We call the revisions "secondary procedures," meaning things we do to improve the appearance when the results are not optimal.

Q: *Let's get specific. What can be done about unsightly insertion scars?*

A: They might be brown or red-brown, indented, or widened. Sometimes that's temporary, but if they persist and are an unacceptable color or have indentations a year after the procedure, we can cut away the skin that is abutting the scar,

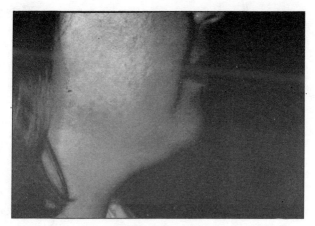

Before neck liposuction

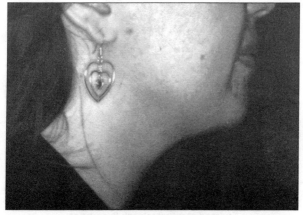

4 months after neck liposuction

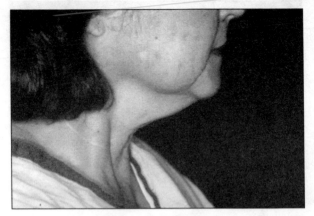

Before neck liposuction

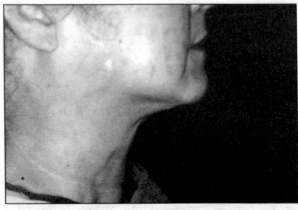

Immediately after neck liposuction

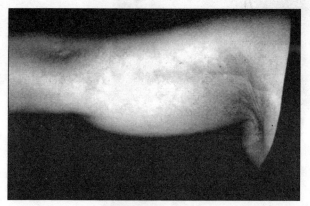

Before upper arm liposuction

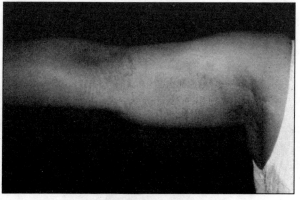

1 week after upper arm liposuction

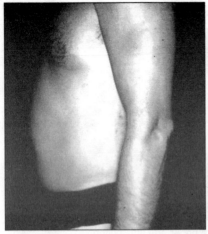

Before breast
(gynecomastia)
liposuction

8 months after
breast liposuction

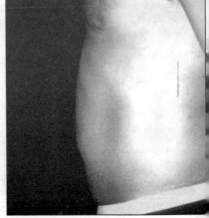

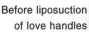
Before liposuction
of love handles

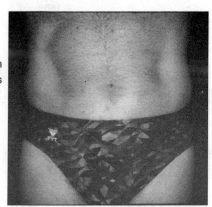

3 weeks
after liposuction
of love handles

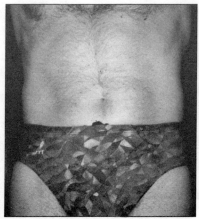

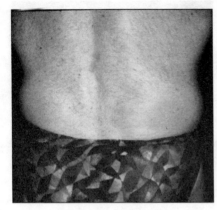

Before liposuction
of love handles

3 weeks after
liposuction
of love handles

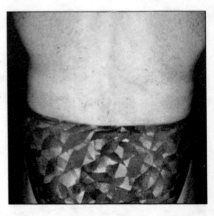

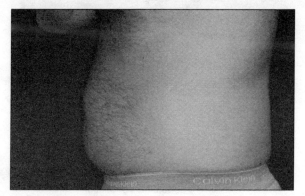

Before abdominal liposuction

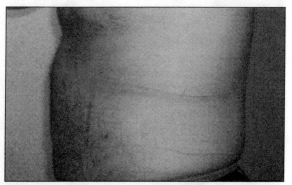

5 days after abdominal liposuction

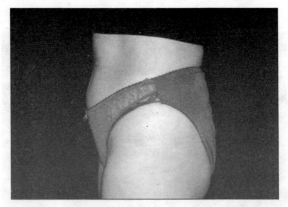

Before abdominal liposuction

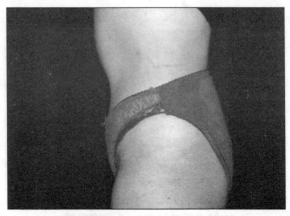

3 months after abdominal liposuction

cut out the scar, then sew it closed to improve it. There is a chance that the new incision might heal in the exact same way—it's just the way that person heals—but in some cases, there is improvement. In any event, they usually look better. We can also use lasers, cortisone, and special dressings to treat problems with scars.

Q: *What can be done about asymmetry?*

A: If it isn't related to the bony framework but is a result of the fat underneath requiring more to be removed from one side, we can go back and do a secondary procedure and get it out. But we have to wait at least six months for the skin to contract from the first liposuction before we do it. This isn't a minor secondary procedure, though; it's like doing the first procedure over again.

Q: *What can be done about skin irregularities?*

A: If the skin has a cellulitelike appearance because patients don't have good skin tone and there is also fat present, external massage can sometimes help. (See Endermologie™ in chapter seventeen.)

Q: *Can anything be done about sensitivity and numbness?*

A: For most people, these tend to improve and go away over time. But there are a few people who have patches of persistent numbness that do not go away. In those cases, people have to learn to live with it. If they have heightened sensitivity, a cream with capsaicin, an over-the-counter red pepper cream, can often be helpful, although it might cause an initial flare of pain upon contact.

Q: *How can swelling, bruising, lumpiness, or hardness be treated?*

A: External ultrasound is wonderful for all of them. The deep penetration of the ultrasound gives a deep massage, helping improve circulation, which in turn gets rid of the bruising and swelling and decreases any lumpiness or hardness in the skin.

Q: *What about significant indentations?*

A: That's something that can be improved by fat injections, whether the area is the size of a thumb print or a hand print. You need more than one treatment, usually three done several months apart. (See Chapter Nineteen for details.)

Q: *What should people know about the cost for secondary procedures?*

A: If a physician knows in advance that liposuction will involve more than one procedure, that will be factored into the total cost. The doctor will tell you, "You're going to have the surgery, then in six months, we will have to do it again." Whether or not you have to pay the equivalent of two separate procedures has to be worked out between you and the doctor. For most physicians, there is a range of fees, but each time a procedure is performed, there are expenses for staff, materials, and sometimes the use of a surgical center of hospital. So it's a good idea to discuss this in advance so you know what to expect.

Q: *We've talked about all kinds of complaints that patients might have, but isn't it a fact that most patients are very happy with their liposuction results?*

A: One recent survey found that after six months, the majority of patients (approximately 98 percent) were satisfied to varying degrees, while only 1 percent were not satisfied. So incidences of people being unhappy with their results and needing additional procedures are actually very rare.

POINTS TO REMEMBER

- There are some areas of resistant fat that might respond to a secondary liposuction procedure.

- Physicians can only remove as much fat as can be taken out safely. Some fat must remain.

- Sometimes patients think too much fat was removed. In such cases, fat injections can often improve results.

- If you are unhappy, bring your complaints directly to your surgeon. Do not consult another doctor first, because your doctor has detailed knowledge about your procedure that no one else has.

- Sometimes people notice areas of their bodies that now seem too big, because another area has been reduced through liposuction and proportions have changed.

- You must wait at least six months for a secondary liposuction procedure.

- There are specific methods for treating most of the problems that patients might have following surgery.

- A recent survey found that only 1 percent of liposuction patients were unhappy with their results, while approximately 98 percent were satisfied.

16
• LIPOSUCTION FOR MEN

ALTHOUGH most liposuction patients are women, the number of men having the surgery is clearly increasing. Current estimates are that approximately 13 percent of patients are men. Most of these men have liposuction on one of two areas: (1) the love handles, which are the fatty bulges along the sides at the waist, and (2) the breasts, which are sometimes enlarged due to a medical condition called "gynecomastia," which means excessive development of the male breast. Men with this condition often suffer many years of self-consciousness, teasing, and harassment. For them, liposuction can be a life changing experience.

In this chapter, we will talk about liposuction procedures for men and what they can accomplish.

Q: *Do you think men are more reluctant to have liposuction than women and when they do, are they more likely to keep it a secret?*

A: In my experience, I haven't found men to be any more reluctant than women to have the surgery or any more concerned with secrecy. I haven't seen any studies on those factors, either. But it might be that fewer men have liposuction because fewer men are aware of it or have knowledge of the details. Women might have learned more about the procedure and understand that it is not for weight loss. Many men continue to believe that if they work out more and watch their diets more carefully, they will be able to get rid of that stubborn pocket of fat—which may in fact be impossible. I say that because many of the men who come in for liposuction are doing crunches, lifting weights, riding bicycles, jogging, swimming, playing basketball, and are generally very active.

Q: *Can you describe the patient who is a good candidate for liposuction of the male breasts?*

A: Typically, he's a man who has noticed he has large breasts, maybe since he's been an adolescent or in his 20s. It's something that's noticed by everyone but rarely spoken about. And it's a big social stigma. Many boys and men with this condition are very self-conscious and don't want to discuss it. They don't want to feel feminized. Eventually, some of them decide to consult a doctor in the hope that something can be done to give them a flatter, more masculine chest.

Q: *What causes this condition?*

A: It can be an endocrine or hormonal imbalance, which stimulates and enlarges the breast tissue in men. Or it can be caused by hereditary factors, obesity, alcoholic cirrhosis, some medications, and certain cancers. Approximately 60 to 70 percent of boys have somewhat enlarged breasts in their teens, but for most, the condition goes away in one to two years. However, studies show that 30 to 40 percent of adult men have some degree of breast enlargement. Even so, we have to ask how much is fat tissue and how much breast tissue? There's no good way for men to test it themselves.

Q: *How can men find out if the enlargement is fatty tissue that can be removed?*

A: They need to be examined by a doctor, either an internist or a plastic surgeon who does both liposuction and surgical procedures for reduction of breast tissue, or a dermatologist. Many dermatologists can perform liposuction, but if the breast tissue has to be resectioned, the patients would probably be referred to a plastic surgeon.

Q: *So men have to find out what condition is causing their breast enlargement first?*

A: Right. Some might have to consult an endocrinologist. They need to have tests to find out if the enlargement is truly a fatty deposit. Once we know it is, then we know we can treat it with liposuction.

Q: *What problems have these men had?*

A: Many of them have had the condition since they were teenagers and have been subjected to ridicule and isolation by their peers. They have suffered from self-consciousness, felt that they had to wear loose shirts to try to hide their condition, and have avoided swimming pools or the beach, where they would have to remove their shirts.

Q: *Is the liposuction surgery to remove fat from male breasts similar to other procedures?*

A: It is more common for male breasts to have firmer, more fibrous fatty tissue that might be more difficult to remove. They have to be in the office for four to five hours, as with most procedures, and that includes preparation time. The procedure itself takes about two and a half to three hours. The surgery requires five insertions—two on each side and one in the middle of the chest.

Q: *How does the patient feel while the surgery is going on?*

A: Once the anesthetic is in and the area is numb, it feels like a massage, but a bit more fibrous than in other areas. Men will feel a gentle to-and-fro motion as the fat is being removed.

Q: *What is the convalescent period like?*

A: Because male breasts are more fibrous and muscular, they tend to bruise more, so compression is very important. A compression garment must be worn. It will minimize bruising, bleeding, and accumulation of blood underneath. Men should also not be very active for the first few weeks. In other words, no benching weights for a while. They should even avoid using their arms for any work for the first few days. They might also have to wait for up to six months to see their final results, because the skin continues to tighten and flatten during that period.

Q: *Are there any unusual side effects that could occur in this area?*

A: There is a small possibility of increased sensitivity or even numbness of the nipple, but it only happens rarely and usually goes away in time.

Q: *How do most men feel after the surgery and convalescence?*

A: More than any other area of liposuction, men undergoing breast reduction wish that more could have been done. Remember, these are often men with very enlarged breasts, and there is only so much fat that can be taken out safely. Even if we're very aggressive, there is an underlying nature of the muscle, and some men have both excess fat and breast tissue. However, these men can get further reduction with plastic surgery.

Despite this, most of the men who have breast reduction liposuction are extremely happy to have visible reduction in an area they thought would remain the same for the rest of their lives. Because of that, we get some of our happiest patients with this procedure, because they have been suffering for such a long time and within one to two days, they see an incredible difference. It's very rewarding surgery for the patient and the medical team.

Q: *The other major area for male liposuction are the love handles. Which men need this surgery?*

A: Very often, they are men who work out and are in good shape all over except in this one area—their "spare tire." These men have good thighs, backs, and stomachs, but they can't get rid of their love handles. Like male breasts, this area also tends to be firmer and more fibrous.

Q: *How does that affect the liposuction procedure?*

A: It means we have to pay attention to using a lot of different-size cannulas as we work to make sure we extract as much fat as we can. We want to be very thorough.

And the love handles are not just on the sides. They actually start in the front, on the sides of the belly, then go up slightly in a diagonal fashion, horizontally across the sides, then back to the midline of the back, going down slowly on an angle. So we have to address all those areas when we perform the surgery.

Q: *Is there anything unusual about this area?*

A: Yes. It's a fatty compartment that is unique to men. And it can make a big difference in a man's contour. Once the fat is removed, it can give a man that V-shape upper torso that is so desirable. Before the surgery, he might not have looked well built in terms of muscular physique in his upper chest area because the love handles were protruding out. But once they're gone, that V-shape is much more obvious and gives the appearance that his upper chest is larger because of the change in proportions. In older men, upper back fat might be resting on the lower love handles and might hang over once the love handles have been done. For these men, liposuction on both the love handles and the back might be recommended.

Q: *How is the convalescent period?*

A: The men have to wear the same compression garments that are used for liposuction on the belly. And if the fat is very fibrous, as in the breasts, there is a chance of more bruising, slightly more discomfort during healing, and swelling that might last longer than it does for women.

Q: *Do men also have liposuction on other areas?*

A: Yes, although they have to be good candidates, of course. Sometimes men have fat removed from their necks, but we have to make sure it is fat, not muscle, and that the result will be in proportion to surrounding areas. Because their skin has a heavier quality, results on men might not be quite as good as those on women. They might also have to wear a compression garment longer to help the skin tighten into position.

Men also have liposuction on the belly. If men have fat above the muscle wall in that area, it can be taken out and they will have a much tighter belly. Liposuction can't be done on a true "beer belly" or "pot belly," because the fat resides behind the muscle wall in those cases. This fat does respond to diet and exercise.

When men have liposuction on the abdomen, more fat can usually be extracted than on women, because male skin is thicker. But the surgeon has to be careful to leave enough fat, because if too much is taken out, the area can develop an irregular mottled-red discoloration from the increased visibility of blood vessels. This is more of a concern for women who undergo aggressive superficial liposuction, because their skin is thinner and can show this discoloration more readily than men.

Those are the more common areas for men, but any of the other areas we address with liposuction can also be done if needed.

POINTS TO REMEMBER

- Approximately 13 percent of liposuction patients are men, with numbers currently increasing.

- Most men have liposuction to reduce enlarged breasts or to reduce love handles.

- It is very likely that fewer men than women know about liposuction and what it can do.

- Enlarged breasts in men have several different causes, and the cause must be found before it is known whether liposuction can be performed.

- Some men need both liposuction and plastic surgery for breast reduction.

- Men who have breast reduction liposuction are usually very happy with the results, although they might wish more could have been removed.

- Men who have liposuction on love handles are often in good shape, exercise regularly, but they just can't get rid of the fat in this area.

- Fat in love handles and male breasts is often firmer and more fibrous, leading to slightly more postsurgical bruising, swelling, and discomfort.

- Men also have liposuction on their necks, bellies, abdomens, and other body areas, but less often than they have it on love handles and breasts.

17

· NEW AND ALTERNATIVE PROCEDURES

IN chapter eight, we talked about the different forms of liposuction that are available for fat removal. As you know, tumescent liposuction is the most frequently performed today, but there are also other, newer types of liposuction procedures and also alternatives to liposuction—other methods for the removal of excess fat. In this chapter, we will talk about some of the newer liposuction procedures and some of the alternatives to liposuction.

Q: *Can you give us a quick review of the history of liposuction?*

A: Liposuction began as a revision of what was earlier attempted by a primitive method to remove fat with a sharp instrument, which caused serious complications. Early liposuction was done with general anesthetic and nontumescent techniques, which caused problems, including a lot of blood loss. Tumescent liposuction, using tumescent anesthetic that allows patients to remain awake and mobile, is now the most commonly performed cosmetic surgical procedure in the country, with a very high safety record.

Q: *What are some of the newer innovations in the field?*

A: Changes in technology allowed the introduction of ultrasonic-assisted liposuction, which, as you recall, can be done internally (although there can be unwanted side effects associated with it) or externally, to soften and liquify the fat. Next came powered liposuction with reciprocating cannulas moving to and fro, making the procedure easier on the surgeon's arm.

Laser-assisted liposuction, like external ultrasound-assisted liposuction, uses noninvasive energy to make the fat looser and somewhat liquid so it's easier to extract. The term doesn't mean that a laser beam is cutting through the skin or entering the fat via a cannula; it means that there is a diode laser with light energy that passes through the skin and heats the tissues below, without damaging the skin. Afterward, tumescent liposuction can be performed, removing the liquified fat.

But this procedure is still investigational, and we don't have long-term results to show whether or not it improves results. The procedure is done with a machine called the Erchonia™ laser. This procedure is similar to externally applied ultrasound, but there is no contact with the skin when using the laser. With ultrasound, the hand piece must contact the skin, creating the risk of a burn if the equipment is left in place and not moved around.

Q: *How is the laser treatment performed?*

A: The treatment lasts for 10 minutes or more and is done prior to liposuction. The laser is held four to six inches away from the body, so it doesn't even touch the skin. The fat becomes emulsified and comes out in a kind of thick, yellowish form, which seems easier for the surgeon to take out. In one study, some patients healed more rapidly and had quicker drainage and less swelling. The study concluded that laser treatment might be a better alternative than external ultrasound to loosen up the fat before doing tumescent liposuction.

Q: *Could this procedure that liquifies fat using laser-assisted liposuction be dangerous?*

A: We don't know. A question arises: Can the external laser liquify fat sufficiently to allow the body to metabolize it without doing the aspiration? There have been no conclusive studies that show that this procedure works.

There is also a medical risk of possible complications when you increase the amount of free fat in the body. For instance, the triglycerides might be taken up by the bloodstream, and if someone has a high content of fat in their blood, they could be at risk for developing some serious conditions, such as pancreatitis. Or the fat could cause blockages that result in a stroke or heart attack. At this point, we don't know.

Q: *Doesn't the external ultrasound-assisted liposuction also liquify fat?*

A: Yes. There are companies that are working on more intensive energy ultrasound to see if the results can be improved.

Q: *What is the treatment that liposuction patients frequently have to smooth out their skin and deal with cellulite following their procedure?*

A: It is called Endermologie™. It was developed in France in the late 1980s and is a nonsurgical treatment designed to condition and contour the skin and reduce the appearance of cellulite. It uses deep-tissue therapeutic massage and gentle suction. Patients have treatments two times a week for one to two months and then go to maintenance treatments once a month. The treatments provide a temporary reduction in cellulite but do not get rid of it permanently. Drinking a lot of water might help produce better results.

Q: *What causes cellulite?*

A: It is thought that cellulite results from swelling of fat and the tension created by fibrous bands between fat lobules.

The bands hold down the skin to the underlying muscle, and when the fat swells, the skin becomes puckered. That happens because the bands hold down the skin like mattress buttons.

Q: *What does the machine look like, and how does it work?*

A: Endermologie™ is a machine with rolling heads, sort of like rolling pins. The unit is also connected to a hose that provides suction to suck up the skin against the rollers. Then the rollers knead the skin. Patients wear a body stocking to decrease the possibility of irritation to their skin.

Q: *Is Endermologie™ always used in conjunction with liposuction?*

A: No. Some patients can get a mild reduction in contour using just the machine, even without liposuction, and sometimes people who don't want to have surgery can get good results using this method. In these cases, the treatment works best for those who need minimal reshaping. In addition, if someone has a lot of irregularity in skin tone, you can try it first to see how they respond to the treatment and get an idea of how much it can help. If patients have irregularities after liposuction, you will already know that Endermologie™ might give them good results.

Endermologie™ also can improve circulation and make tissues softer for liposuction patients.

Q: *How long after liposuction do people have Endermologie™, and how much does it cost?*

A: They usually have it about a month after surgery, and each session costs in the neighborhood of $100.

Q: *Tell us about injections to dissolve fat.*

A: That is another investigational type of procedure using two chemicals that are in the process of being studied. One is phosphatidyl choline, and the other is collagenase. The concerns are similar to those involving external ultrasound or laser liposuction. What happens when fat is liquified in the body? We need more studies to find out, because there could be dangerous side effects or long-term problems. So we will have to wait for future results.

POINTS TO REMEMBER

- Ultrasonic-assisted liposuction can be done internally, although there can be unwanted side effects, and externally to liquify fat.

- Laser-assisted liposuction uses noninvasive energy to loosen and soften fat. The diode laser does not actually touch the body or affect the skin.

- Laser-assisted liposuction is still investigational and might have unknown risks.

- Endermologie™ can smooth skin and improve cellulite after liposuction. Used alone, it can improve skin condition and contour through deep massage and gentle suction.

• Researchers are studying two chemicals that may, in the future, be injected to dissolve fat, if they are found to be safe and effective.

18

· OTHER MEDICAL USES FOR LIPOSUCTION

SO far, we have talked about how cosmetic liposuction techniques are used to remove excess fat from various parts of the body to recontour your shape and make it more attractive. But liposuction can do more than just improve the appearance of your body. It can also be used for removing fatty deposits and growths caused by certain medical conditions. In this chapter, we will look at some of the other medical uses for liposuction.

Q: *In addition to fat removal and recontouring, what other medical uses does liposuction have?*

A: Liposuction can be used for the removal of lipomas and hematomas, insulin-induced fat deposits, and fat accumulations due to Madelung's disease; to treat excessive sweating;

and for breast reduction in women (which we do not recommend).

Q: *What are lipomas, and how is liposuction used to remove them?*

A: Lipomas are fatty growths that can occur in lumps underneath the skin. They vary in size and can be from a half-inch to ten inches in diameter. Instead of having to make a long incision to remove a large lipoma, which would leave a long scar, liposuction can reduce or sometimes remove them using very small insertion areas.

Q: *Can liposuction remove the entire lipoma?*

A: Probably not, especially if it is large. These fatty growths are actually benign tumors, and they also tend to get bigger. Surgeons will try to remove all the lipoma, but some remnants are usually left behind and can grow in the future. So it is likely that surgical removal would be more effective, but even so, liposuction is still used to deal with lipomas.

Q: *How is liposuction used to remove other fat deposits?*

A: There is an inherited disease called Madelung's disease, which is characterized by deposits of fat in significant volumes located in different parts of the body. One of the more common areas is the lower neck and the upper back. That area can also get fatty from people who take long-term medical steroids for diseases like arthritis and lupus.

These areas can be treated with liposuction, which is a very practical solution for people who are bothered by such fat deposits. But we have to be certain that the procedure will be completely safe for these patients, so a medical clearance is very important.

Q: *How is liposuction used to treat excessive sweating?*

A: In the past, liposuction was used in the underarm area through a small insertion to try to go underneath the skin. The idea was not so much to remove fat as to scrape the underneath of the skin, the dermis, where the sweat glands reside. Because if you remove the gland, there will be a lot less sweating. Today, however, that treatment is not commonly done because Botox is used instead.

There is another treatment for this condition in which skin is actually cut out of the underarm area, leaving skin that has fewer sweat glands, but the procedure also leaves a long scar that can get raised and irritated.

Q: *How is liposuction used to treat hematomas?*

A: If someone develops a hematoma from surgery—liposuction or any other kind of surgery—it is possible to use liposuction to extract the hematoma. We already talked about using a needle to extract the liquid in the hematoma once it liquifies, but you can also use liposuction, while the hematoma is clotted, to get it out.

So if the hematoma is large and the person is bothered by it, it can be taken out with liposuction. But there is one caution: Surgeons have to realize that although they can perform liposuction to remove the clot, the procedure might cause another hematoma to form.

Q: *How is liposuction used for reconstructive surgery?*

A: Sometimes there is too much skin and fat. Let's say a skin cancer has been removed and there is a flap of skin to cover the hole. After this procedure, the area might heal nicely, but sometimes it remains thick. Liposuction can sometimes be used to take out fat from the flap or the surrounding area and smooth things out.

POINTS TO REMEMBER

- Although liposuction is used mainly to remove excess fat for cosmetic purposes, it has other medical uses.

- Liposuction can remove or reduce lipomas, fatty growths under the skin that can be of varying sizes.

- Madelung's disease and long-term use of medical steroids can also cause large fat deposits, which can be taken out using liposuction.

- Excessive sweating has been treated in the past with liposuction, but today, Botox is usually the preferred treatment.

- Clotted hematomas from surgery can be removed using liposuction, but the procedure might sometimes create another hematoma.

- Liposuction can be used to make areas of reconstructive surgery more even and smooth through the removal of excess fat.

19

• FAT INJECTIONS

ALTHOUGH the use of fat injections is a separate procedure from liposuction, they are often used together. This process allows the surgeon to make good use of the fat that is being removed during liposuction—or as I often like to say, "waist not, want not." It also allows the patient to begin the procedure of having indentations and depressions filled in at the same time excess fat is being taken out. Using your own fat as a filler has many advantages. In this chapter, we will explain how fat injections work, why they are often used in conjunction with liposuction, and what kinds of results you can anticipate.

Q: *What are fat injections?*

A: They are injections of a person's own fat that is removed from some part of the body and put into another part, where it acts as a filler.

Q: *Why do people need fat injections?*

A: Fat is a filler used to restore volume reduction, including visible indentations and depressions in the skin. These types of volume reduction can occur with weight loss and the aging process. It makes the typical face look tired, ill, and sagging, even when the person doesn't feel that way.

Q: *What are the typical areas for fat injections?*

A: The areas most patients want treated are the smile folds that extend from the corner of the nostrils diagonally down the face to the corners of the lips and then sometimes down to the chin. Many people also want fillers on their lips to enlarge them. Lips might be thin to begin with or might become thinner with aging.

The hollows of the cheeks are another popular area for fillers. They can occur because of heredity, with significant weight loss, or as a side effect of some medications.

Fat can also be injected in the temples when they develop an unhealthy-looking hollowness; to fill in and raise the eyebrow area when it is lowered; to make the area around the eyes smoother in contour and more youthful; for chin augmentation in people who have small chins, and also for the forehead, upper and lower eyelids, cheekbones, and jawline. Fat can also be used to fill in depressions from automobile accidents, skin cancer, and even from liposuction.

Q: *Can it be used on all indentations and depressions?*

A: No. If someone has only superficial lines and fine creases, they are not a candidate for fat injections, because fat is at a deeper layer. We don't use fat within the skin layer itself; we implant it between the skin and the fat layers. So it's great for deep smile folds, but not for tiny lines. It can also be very risky to use it around the eyes and between the eyebrows, so you have to be very careful when working in those areas.

Q: *What other fillers are used?*

A: Collagen is the most common treatment. There is collagen from cows and human collagen, which is purified. There are also newer fillers such as Artecoll, which was recently approved by the FDA. There's also Gortex, a permanent, synthetic implant, that many people like. If they don't like it, it can be removed. There are also investigational substances. The big worry with the newer substances is the possibility of side effects or complications that could occur over time.

Q: *Are there any problems with using collagen?*

A: Cow collagen can be a very expensive filler, especially if there is a large area to treat. Collagen doesn't last long.

It's usually resorbed in two to six months and then you need to get more injections. It never lasts forever. There are also people who are allergic to cow collagen, which can't happen with your own fat. You have to take two skin tests before you can use collagen. There are some people who do not like the idea of using human collagen from another person and prefer their own fat.

Q: *Do you use collagen as a filler for areas that could be treated with fat?*

A: If people come to me asking for treatment on deep smile folds, I encourage them to try collagen first to see if they like the results. If they don't like the way it looks, then they will not have to go through the procedure of having to harvest fat from their body and implant it.

Q: *Is there a perfect filler?*

A: We are still searching for one. It would be something easy to use that creates a smooth feel and natural appearance, doesn't cause pain, is inexpensive, is permanent, doesn't move or shift, doesn't create irregularities or infections, and has no risk of allergic reactions.

Q: *Does your own fat have significant advantages over collagen?*

A: It can save certain patients a lot of money, depending on how much collagen they need, because fat injections can be retained as a permanent graft on a long-term basis. When that happens, patients don't have to keep coming back to get more fillers every few months. But it doesn't happen for everyone. In some patients, none of the fat is retained, so we have variable results. We just have to wait and see how each patient responds.

When your own fat is injected, it also feels more natural. Collagen is a little firmer.

Q: *If all the fat from the first treatment is resorbed, does that mean the same thing will happen with additional treatments?*

A: No, absolutely not. There are many patients who had no retention of the fat from the first treatment and have had retention on further treatments.

Q: *How are fat injections connected to liposuction?*

A: Because fat is removed during liposuction, if you need a filler, you can make immediate use of that fat to begin working on the area that needs filling.

Q: *How many treatments are required?*

A: There is more than one treatment. Usually, it involves three to five treatments, which I do several months apart. I believe it's important to give the injected fat a chance to take root and develop new circulation. Depending on the situation, we might wait anywhere from three to nine months between treatments.

Q: *How much of the fat takes root?*

A: That depends on the patient. Some of it is going to be resorbed and will not take root because the body doesn't allow 100 percent of new cells placed in it to live. So the second procedure builds on the first, and the third builds on the second.

Q: *Can you describe the procedure?*

A: If patients have liposuction, we are able to use the fat that is being removed during the procedure. This fat comes out yellow, but it still has anesthetic in it, which must be taken out. We put the fat in a centrifuge using a sterile technique, and it is briefly spun to remove the anesthetic liquid and some oils. We usually inject it before we continue with the liposuction procedure, so the fat is fresh when it's implanted. Sometimes, it can be put in after the liposuction procedure has been done.

For people who are not undergoing liposuction, we find some fat in an area where it can be removed safely and put it in the centrifuge to prepare it. Usually, it comes from the upper buttock area or the belly, but sometimes from the outer thigh, because as we know these are areas where the fat does not go away with diet and exercise. So we are taking resistant fat that will have a greater chance of being retained when we implant it in a different area. Then, with local anesthetic, we make a very tiny opening in the area where the fat is going to be implanted. Using a little cannula, we get into different areas and insert the fat.

Q: *Can this procedure be done on everyone?*

A: Pretty much, but there could be problems with very thin people who had liposuction on their last deposit of excess fat, making it difficult to find the extra fat to harvest.

Q: *How long does the procedure take?*

A: It's very straightforward, but it does take from 45 minutes to an hour in the office.

Q: *Is there any pain?*

A: The removal of the fat is not painful at all. When we inject the fat, we have to put in a local anesthetic, which might sting a little bit. In the lip area, the procedure can be uncomfortable, so some patients need local anesthetic and numbing cream.

Q: *Are there any side effects?*

A: Some people have swelling for day or two, so you shouldn't have the procedure the day before a big social event. There can also be bruising and sometimes lumpiness or other irregularities. But many people look fine the next day. They don't need a big dressing, just a little bit of tape. Infections are very rare.

Q: *How long do patients have to be away from work?*

A: About three days—sometimes less and rarely more.

Q: *If you have liposuction and the removed fat is used for the first treatment, is the remainder frozen for future treatments?*

A: There are two schools of thought on that. Those in favor of freezing believe it makes it easier for patients, because you won't have to put them through the fat removal procedure a second time. Others, like me, who are not in favor of freezing, remove the fat needed for injection during each treatment.

Q: *Are there any long-term concerns about fat injections?*

A: When you implant your own fat, there are not any concerns about the possibility of systemic illness brought about by an immune response to a foreign substance. We feel confident that even many years after fat injections, it's unlikely that any growths or hard lumpiness would develop that would have to be removed. Of course, it is possible that fatty cysts can develop and create lumps, and some lumpiness can occur after the injections, but they are normally very small areas and can be extracted.

Q: *Do doctors need special training to perform fat injections?*

A: Yes. You have to ask your doctor about it. The procedure is really quite complicated, and experience is important.

Q: *How much do fat injections cost?*

A: Costs will vary according to where you live, your doctor, whether the fat is taken fresh for each treatment or frozen, how many times you have to come for treatment, and how much is being implanted. An average cost would be from $1,200 to several thousand dollars.

Q: *How would you summarize the benefits of fat injections?*

A: If someone has depressions or if they just have an aged appearance, fat is a very nice alternative to other fillers. If you're going to have it removed with liposuction anyway, why not recycle it and use it to improve these areas?

POINTS TO REMEMBER

- Patients can use fat that has been removed during liposuction for injections to fill indentations or depressions in various parts of the body.

- Areas where fillers are frequently used include smile folds, lips, cheeks, temples, eyebrows, chins, and around the eyes.

- Fat injections work on deep depressions, not superficial lines and creases.

- Fat can be a good alternative to collagen and has several advantages over it.

- From three to five fat injection treatments are administered several months apart.

- In the best cases, some of the fat takes root and becomes permanent, although this doesn't happen for everyone.

- Some doctors freeze fat for future treatments; others remove the fat each time and use it fresh.

- Doctors need special training and experience to perform fat injections.

20

• TAKING CARE OF YOURSELF BEFORE AND AFTER LIPOSUCTION

BY now, you have learned the most important facts about liposuction: It is not a treatment for weight loss; it is a method for removing stubborn fat deposits that won't come off with diet and exercise; and the best candidates are people who eat well, exercise regularly, and are at their ideal weight or only slightly over. Because of this, people who want liposuction for weight loss are often turned away by doctors, with the advice to change their diets, maintain an exercise program, and come back in six months or longer.

But what is a healthy diet? What kind of exercise do you need, and how often do you have to do it? What else can you do to stay healthy? And if you are a good liposuction candidate and are planning to have the procedure, how can you take care of yourself before and after the procedure to maximize your chances for great results? In this chapter, we will find out exactly what Dr. Shelton advises.

Q: *What is one important thing patients can do prior to liposuction to maximize their chances of getting good results?*

A: Quit smoking. You should stop smoking in general, for overall health improvement. But if you don't want to, you should at least abstain from smoking for two weeks before and one week after surgery. Remember that smoking robs the bloodstream of oxygen, and you need oxygen to heal. Smoking also contains toxins, and nicotine clamps down on your blood vessels and constricts them. That could increase your blood pressure and also your risk of bleeding. Smoking also has many negative effects on the skin, causing wrinkles and other signs of premature aging. So there are many reasons to stop smoking.

Q: *What about secondhand smoke?*

A: That is also bad. You don't want to be breathing smoke from other smokers around you. You should also realize that if you are smoking a pipe or cigar and not inhaling, you are still getting secondhand smoke. And smoking includes marijuana. The bottom line is, do not smoke if you want good liposuction results.

Q: *What else should people avoid?*

A: Alcohol, which makes people bleed more. I recommend that people abstain from alcoholic drinks for a few days before and at least a day after the procedure. Alcohol is also metabolized by the liver, and if someone has a lot to drink a day before liposuction, the liver is still processing the alcohol and might not be able to process the anesthetic as well.

Q: *What about your diet?*

A: No crash diets! If you've been told by your doctor that you should lose a little more weight to get better results from liposuction, you should never go on a crash diet to try to lose the weight quickly. When you do that, you can go into a protein-wasting state and some of your muscle mass can begin to degrade. The more protein you lose, the less well you will heal. You body needs to produce collagen and you need good protein stores to heal properly.

Q: *What makes up a good diet?*

A: You should have a balance of roughly one third of your calories from each of three groups: proteins, carbohydrates, and fats.

Q: *How much water do people need to drink?*

A: Patients don't need a lot of extra water, but they should not be dehydrated. If they are drinking the average amount of water, about six to eight 8-ounce glasses a day (which includes beverages made with water), that should be fine. If they are not getting enough liquids and are dehydrated, the body will not heal as well. Blood pressure might be low and you can have dizziness when you stand up after surgery. And if the blood pressure falls too low, we might not even be able to perform the procedure.

Q: *What about the use of caffeine?*

A: It depends on how much you consume. It's not a good idea to have a heart rate increase based on caffeine consumption when you are undergoing liposuction, because the adrenaline in the anesthetic could raise your pulse significantly and cause a problem during the procedure. But for most people, drinking one or two cups of coffee, tea, or caffeinated soda a day, including the day before surgery, would be all right. More than that is probably not good because caffeine is a diuretic, meaning that it makes you urinate more often and you can begin to dehydrate. So keep your caffeine consumption from moderate to none around the time of liposuction.

Q: *Is it a good idea for people to take vitamin supplements?*

A: Certain vitamins can be beneficial for general health and for dealing with surgery. The risks of megadosing are not well understood, but you should have at least the minimum daily requirements of most vitamins and minerals. That's why I recommend a daily multivitamin and a multivitamin with iron for most women. If you are deficient in vitamin C, you can have problems with collagen production. You also want to make sure you have enough calcium, vitamin B complex for healthy nerves, and vitamin A, which also helps with collagen production.

Q: *Are there any other substances that people can take to help with surgery?*

A: Many patients ask about taking some alternative medications, such as Arnica Montana (see chapter nine) and bromelain. Bromelain is an enzyme that some people find helpful for healing minor injuries; they claim it reduces swelling, bruising, pain, and tenderness. But bromelain is also a blood thinner, so it must be taken in the right amount under medical supervision. Some people also experience allergic reactions or side effects, so great care should be taken in using this substance.

There are also reports that Arnica can be toxic to the heart if taken in high doses. So although there are lots of positive anecdotal reports on the use of these two substances, the medical jury is still out. If you want to try them, consult your physician first.

Q: *Are there any other substances people should avoid?*

A: Earlier, we mentioned staying away from grapefruit, because it interferes with the action of the anesthetic. Also avoid vitamin E, because it can cause bleeding. You should also abstain from any illicit drugs, including cocaine, which can cause stimulation of the heart and add greatly to the risks of liposuction surgery.

Q: *How can exposure to the sun or tanning parlors affect liposuction results?*

A: If you have a blistering sunburn, you will not be able to have surgery. If you get a tan without blistering, your skin will be peeling after liposuction, and you might be very uncomfortable with your compression garment on. So you should avoid tanning parlors or sunbathing prior to liposuction.

Afterward, you will also want to avoid them for a while because you don't want the insertion scars to get dark. And remember that a suntan is never a healthy thing anyway because of the risks of skin cancer and premature aging.

Q: *Are there any special creams or lotions that can help with healing?*

A: You want to keep the insertion sites moist, but you are given antibiotic ointment for that purpose. Other creams such as aloe vera might also help. Some people use vitamin E creams, but there is no scientific evidence that these promote healing.

It's also important to know that both aloe vera and vitamin E are sensitizers, meaning that they are composed of chemicals that can, over repeated use, eventually sensitize your skin, causing an allergic reaction. In addition, there is really no need for these creams.

Q: *Is an exercise program beneficial for liposuction patients?*

A: Definitely. Prior to liposuction, it's essential. Patients should resume exercising shortly after the procedure. Anyone who has been exercising regularly has better circulation, is usually better rested, and has a better frame of mind to cope with the stresses during and after surgery. If someone isn't working out regularly, they might find it takes them longer to heal, because their circulation is not working as effectively. So exercise is a wonderful help to our bodies on many different levels and is a big plus for responding well to surgery.

Q: *When can people go back to exercise after the procedure?*

A: Most people can return to the gym within a few days to a week, but it should not be overly aggressive exercise. Moderate exercise helps your body heal quicker because you are moving around and you won't form adhesions and build up scar material the way you could if you're just sitting around and watching television and not moving.

Q: *Is your emotional state important?*

A: In general, people with positive attitudes tend to recover more quickly, while those with negative attitudes might obsess about everything and not focus on how they are healing and getting better. They might even begin to imagine symptoms that aren't there, increasing their stress and making it harder to heal.

For instance, the soreness after liposuction is like the soreness you feel after a hard work out at the gym. In other words, it's not so bad and soon gets better. If you have a negative attitude, you tend to concentrate on what's bad and exaggerate it in your mind, making it worse. But if you have a positive attitude, you might not even notice that a buttock is sore when you sit down the second day after surgery. Then days go by, and all of a sudden you realize nothing hurts anymore.

Q: *How can everyday stress affect your results?*

A: People who are under stress tend to feel pain more, because their whole central nervous system is hypersensitive. It's similar to sleep deprivation, which stressed people can experience as well.

It's important to be well rested for your procedure. The more relaxed you are, the more at ease you are, and the more positive your attitude is about getting good results, the better you're going to do during surgery, the better you are going to heal, and the happier you're going to be.

Lack of proper rest can also occur when patients fly in from out of town, feel exhausted from jet lag, and come directly for surgery. It's always better if, when you are traveling a distance, to give yourself an extra day to rest prior to surgery.

POINTS TO REMEMBER

- Do not smoke for two weeks prior to and one week following liposuction. Also avoid secondhand smoke.

- Don't drink alcohol for a few days before and after your procedure.

- Don't use crash diets to lose weight to qualify for liposuction.

- Be sure to drink enough fluids so you don't become dehydrated.

- Use caffeine in moderation prior to and after surgery.

- A daily multivitamin is recommended.

- Avoid sun exposure, because a tan or blisters can affect or even cancel your procedure.

- Regular exercise promotes good circulation and faster healing.

- People with positive attitudes usually heal better and often have better results.

- Be well rested on the day you have liposuction.

21

• CASE HISTORIES

IN the following case histories, names and other identifying characteristics have been changed to protect the privacy of the patients. In some instances, composites have been created for the purposes of illustration. All the medical facts are accurate.

Remember that all these case histories involve individual, unique cases. No two people are alike, and no two people will respond in the exact same way to liposuction. These case histories are intended as informative examples and are not intended as a guide to how you might respond to liposuction surgery.

Peggy: No More Sagging Neck

A 59-year-old college professor, Peggy had been very unhappy with her sagging neck for some time. But when she came in, she explained that she didn't want to have a surgical neck-lift. She asked if there was anything else that could help improve her appearance. Peggy had slight loosening of her neck muscle, but most of her sagging was due to excess fat tissue. I recommended liposuction, and despite the wrinkling in her skin, the results were quite good. Now, Peggy is very pleased with the results of her surgery.

Claudia: Let's do it again

Claudia was a 40-year-old Internet executive who had undergone a surgical breast reduction and liposuction on her thighs several years before she came to see me. Now, Claudia wanted to know if she could reduce her lower abdomen, because she had discovered that years of working out had no effect on the fat in that area. Claudia was healthy and close to her ideal weight. We performed tumescent liposuction and removed about half a liter of fat. With very little discomfort, Claudia was able to return to work in three days. However, she noticed puffiness in a small area of her lower belly about two weeks later, which we treated with external ultrasound. A week later, Claudia was much improved and now that she has healed completely, she is extremely happy with her results.

Elinor: It runs in the family

Thirty-year-old Elinor, a dental assistant, explained that all the women in her family had large legs. She had liposuction in my office on her outer thighs, hips, and inner knees and was very surprised that the procedure was painless. Six months later, Elinor returned for another liposuction procedure. This time she wanted more fat removed from the fronts of her thighs. For the second procedure, Elinor said she felt some pain, but when she returned a few months later, she was very happy with her flatter thighs. Although Elinor is pleased with her procedures, she is still interested in removing more fat from her legs and is now considering an additional liposuction procedure.

Walter: A Flatter Chest at Last

A 52-year-old investment banker, Walter told me that he had enlarged breasts since his early 20s and had been trying to reduce them with dieting and exercise, without any good results. Walter had tumescent liposuction, and once the fat was removed, his chest was immediately flatter. Fat was also removed from around his nipples so the contour of his chest would be smooth. Walter found that his chest was a little sore for a day after surgery, describing the feeling as "like after a good workout with weights." There was only slight swelling, and Walter returned to work in two days and went back to the gym in four. After three months, Walter found that he was no longer self-conscious about his chest and felt much more comfortable in clothes.

Lori: No Excess Fat

A 26-year-old graduate student, Lori seemed very nervous when she came in for her consultation. She explained that she was studying for her finals but wanted to make an appointment for liposuction on her thighs so she could look good for the summer. After examining her, I told Lori that she was in very good shape and had no excess fat that could be removed. She kept pinching her right thigh and insisting that there were ugly lumps that she had to get rid of right away. Realizing that Lori did not have a realistic image of her body, I explained the liposuction procedure to her and demonstrated that the small amount of fat she had in her thighs was needed and could not be removed. When she refused to accept my diagnosis, I gently suggested that Lori might be under a lot of pressure and should think about counseling. Three months later, I was very surprised to receive a phone call from her thanking me for my honesty and advice. "A lot of doctors would have operated anyway," she said. "You were right. I was really stressed out, and I'm getting some help now. I really have to thank you."

Naomi: A More Beautiful Neck

Naomi was a 31-year-old administrative assistant who had been bothered by her full neck since adolescence. "It's just like my mother's," she told me. She had tried diet and exercise to reduce the size of her neck, but nothing worked. Although she was slightly overweight all over her body, she was concerned about her neck because it was so visible to everyone. She turned out to be a good candidate for neck liposuction, and the procedure went very smoothly. However, following surgery, Naomi developed some swelling, bleeding, and a hematoma. After treating the hematoma, we saw that it had become smaller and softer.

Four months later, the hematoma was gone and Naomi was completely healed, extremely pleased with her new appearance.

Gwendolyn: Fat Rolls on the Back

Gwendolyn, a 51-year-old chef, was at her ideal body weight but did not exercise regularly. She was unhappy with the rolls of fat on her back under her bra straps. When I examined this area, I found that the fat was rather firm and fibrous, so I informed her that the improvement might be less than she wanted. Gwendolyn decided to have liposuction anyway, explaining that "any improvement will be better than what I have now."

Two weeks after the procedure, Gwendolyn's results looked very smooth, but she still had some swelling. After a month, it became evident that Gwendolyn's skin had reformed some of the rolls, which is not unusual in this area. The appearance was certainly better than before surgery, but it was not perfect, partly due to her naturally sagging skin. Gwendolyn said she was somewhat satisfied with the results, but wished she had fewer rolls on her back. However, she understood that these rolls were mostly related to her sagging skin, and she was still glad she had undergone the surgery, even though she didn't achieve everything she had hoped for.

Tricia: Extra Fat on the Belly

Tricia, a 44-year-old lawyer, explained that her mother, sisters, and grandmother all had a tendency to put on weight on their lower bellies and, she explained, "now it's happening to me." During the consultation, I found that Tricia had an inch of fat on her lower belly that could be pinched between the fingers. She also had excess fat on her lower buttocks, which pushed on the outer thighs, causing the false impression of fatty thighs—what is called "pseudo saddlebags." I recommended buttock liposuction, but Tricia wanted only abdominal liposuction. A small amount of fat was removed during the abdominal procedure, including some from the area around her belly button. Tricia recovered quickly, with no bruising and only a little discomfort. She told me, "I love the way I look now."

Simon: Getting Rid of Love Handles

Bothered by his love handles for many years, Simon, a 55-year-old landscape gardener, was in good overall shape. He worked out for an hour every day and ate a healthy diet, but the small amount of bulging fat at his love handles simply would not come off. "If I get this fixed," he told me, "I think my body will finally look the way I want it to." Simon had tumescent liposuction and saw an immediate improvement, as fat was removed from each side of his body. Although he had some bruising and numbness, Simon went back to the gym in a few days and said that the more he exercised, the better he felt. Simon's results have remained excellent, and when he was contacted by our office four years later, he reported that, "I'd rate my surgery an 11 out of 10. That's how happy I am when I look in the mirror every day."

Janice: Too Much

When Janice, a 44-year-old emergency room nurse, came to see me, she was about 60 pounds overweight. She explained that she had very active job and got a lot of exercise at work, but she just couldn't get rid of her extra fat. After examining her and talking with her, I told Janice it would not be a good idea to do liposuction now, because she had generalized excess weight, not small concentrated areas of extra fat. We reviewed her diet and physical exercise, and Janice realized that she was not eating as healthy a diet as she imagined and that her physical exercise at work was not sufficient to remove the fat she kept adding through poor food choices. I advised Janice to follow a recommended diet and exercise program and come back in six months to a year, or whenever she had lost at least 40 pounds. I cautioned her not to go on a crash diet and to be certain to lose the weight slowly and sensibly. Two years later, Janice returned, having lost 50 pounds. She was very proud of her accomplishment and looked like a different person. "I'm ready for my liposuction, doctor," she told me. Janice had liposuction in two separate procedures on her outer thighs, buttocks, and upper back. With her weight loss and new contour, Janice was extremely pleased, and three years later, she has continued to maintain her weight.

Crystal: Asymmetric Thighs

A kindergarten teacher, Crystal was a 39-year-old woman who was very health-conscious, ate well, and worked out at the gym on a regular basis. Her problem was her outer thighs, which had extra fat that she could not work off. In addition, the thighs were of different sizes, one heavier than the other. "My mother had the same problem," she told me. Unhappy with the excess fat and lack of symmetry in her outer thighs, Crystal decided to have liposuction. A large amount of fat was removed from Crystal's outer thighs, more from the larger right thigh than the smaller left thigh. The minute Crystal stood up after the procedure and saw that her thighs were now the same size and nicely contoured, tears of joy came into her eyes and she thanked our medical team for finally making her dream come true.

Monique: Great in a Miniskirt

As an editor for a women's fashion magazine, 35-year-old Monique liked to wear the latest styles, including some very short skirts. But because of unwanted fat deposits on her lower abdomen and inner knees, Monique was often self-conscious. "I feel as though all the other women are looking at me and feeling sorry for me," she commented. Although Monique exercised regularly at her aerobics class and was close to her ideal weight, the fat deposits on her lower abdomen and inner knees would not budge. Monique was very happy when she realized that liposuction could be the answer, and she had the procedure soon after her consultation. She was able to return to work in a few days, reporting that she had very little discomfort, but did not like wearing the compression garment. Now, two years later, Monique reports that she is very happy with her results and no longer worries about what her co-workers think when she wears revealing outfits.

Anthony: Taking Time to Decide

Anthony, a 29-year-old architect, told me that he had been thinking about liposuction for about 5 years. He explained that he was a chubby child and an overweight adolescent, but in his early 20s, he decided to take better care of himself. Losing 60 pounds, eating better, and working out regularly, Anthony had sculpted his body so it was almost exactly what he wanted. But he couldn't get rid of his love handles, no matter how much time he spent at the gym. Anthony told me, "I don't like the idea of surgery, but I read a lot about it and decided that this was my only solution." The procedure to remove excess fat from Anthony's love handles went very well, and a good amount of fat came out. Three days later, Anthony was back at work, and a week later, he was back in the gym. He reported that a lot of people commented on how good he looked, but no one realized why. Now, he's telling some of his male friends and encouraging them to think about liposuction for their love handles.

Opal: Never Too Late

Although she was 66 years old, Opal had always taken good care of herself, had good genes, and looked at least 10 years younger. Her skin had good elasticity and tone,

and she was a good liposuction candidate for removal of
the love handles that had bothered her for so long. "I've
had other procedures," she told me, "but never liposuction.
I'd really like to get rid of that ugly fat on my sides and
stop worrying about how it looks to everyone." Opal's surgery went very smoothly, and she was extremely pleased
with her new shape. "After all these years," she told us,
"those horrible bulges are really gone. It's a miracle!"

22

• CONCLUSION

BY now, you have learned a great deal about liposuction—maybe even more than you want or need to know. But it's all for the good, because the better informed you are about any medical procedure you undergo, the better your results can be. In this chapter, we will return to some of the most important points in this book and try to give you a clear and concise picture of the liposuction procedure and what it can do for you.

Q: *Can almost anyone benefit from liposuction?*

A: No. If they have a generalized increased amount of fat, then liposuction in one area will not give them a more attractive appearance. In fact, it could make their bodies look out of proportion. If people are generally over-weight, the chances are they are not eating properly and exercising regularly, so it is quite possible that you will perform liposuction and they will regain the weight. And then there are people who are thin and don't have any accumulations of fat that need to be removed, so they are not candidates.

Q: *Do many people have the wrong ideas about liposuction?*

A: Definitely. There's a widespread idea that if you are overweight, liposuction is an easy way to get rid of the fat. These people don't realize that liposuction is not a weight loss treatment, but a way for people to recontour their bodies by removing small pockets of fat that they can't get rid of through diet and exercise.

There are also many people who say, "Who needs liposuction? Why don't those people just diet and exercise more?" Again, they don't realize that no matter how much people diet and exercise, there are certain areas where fat accumulates and will not go down. Many of these people had just one momentary lapse in their lives when they gained weight and now they can't shed it in that one area. They just can't get it off.

Many people also falsely believe that liposuction is a very painful procedure. They've seen the early demonstrations on television that were pretty unpleasant to watch, and they don't know that for almost every patient, the procedure is not painful at all. They've also heard some frightening stories about bad results from early procedures and don't realize that with the newer tumescent procedure, there is an excellent safety record.

People also assume that they are going to have to stay

home for weeks to recuperate, when in reality, most people are back at work in a few days.

Q: *Can liposuction have a dramatic effect on people who are good candidates?*

A: I just saw a patient recently who told me, "Liposuction changed my life." Even I was surprised to hear that. It turned out that he was so happy to get rid of his love handles, which he had been trying to exercise down for years, that he became very health-conscious. He stopped smoking, changed his diet, and developed a much more positive attitude about everything.

Q: *Do you think liposuction will continue to grow in popularity?*

A: Yes, I do. Several years ago, there was a resurgence in liposuction. One of the reasons is the development of tumescent liposuction, which is extremely safe and does not require hospitalization or a lot of down time. Remember that it is the most popular cosmetic surgical procedure performed in this country. With increased health information so widely available through the media and Internet, more and more people are learning about it. I also don't see any alternative treatments on the horizon that will be as safe or effective. I'm sure there will be some in the future, but I don't think they will be available in the next few years.

Q: *Why do you think it's important for patients to be well informed?*

A: In my office, we work as a team, and I have always found that a well-informed patient helps the team. Medicine can't be rendered well without active participation on the part of patients. Patients need to understand the procedure they will undergo, its benefits and risks, and understand what they will experience before, during, and after surgery. They should know when to call the doctor, what to tell the doctor, and what questions to ask. The more they understand in advance, the calmer they will be during the entire procedure. Lack of knowledge can often cause stress, anxiety, and fear, which are never beneficial when it comes to health care.

Finally, when patients understand exactly what is going on with their care, they will realize they are not just going through a procedure and that's it. They will know that good health is a lifelong commitment, and they will make that commitment to keep themselves healthy—not just for a few weeks or months, or a year, but permanently.

Q: *Can you summarize the major benefits and drawbacks of liposuction?*

A: The major benefit is that if you are an appropriate candidate, you can not only lose the amount of fat you are unhappy with—the fat you tried to reduce for many years—you can also see it go away in a matter of a couple hours. Long-term results are very good, with a fewer than 1 percent complication rate for tumescent liposuction. Also, people in their 50s and 60s and even beyond are possible candidates, whereas they were not with the older technique. And the recovery period is rather short. Finally, studies show an excellent satisfaction rate, up to 98 percent, with more than 50 percent indicating very high satisfaction.

The drawbacks? One is the time that you have to take off from work, although for most people, it's only a few days. There's the cost of the procedure; the discomfort, swelling, and bruising most people experience during convalescence; the need to wear compression garments; limitations to activity for a few days to weeks; and the possibility of having to use your vacation time for the procedure.

Liposuction is a great procedure. It's not for everyone, and the results can't be guaranteed. But when it works well, which is most of the time, people are often ecstatic about their new shapes. Many of them a report significant increase in self-confidence and self-esteem and wonder why in the world they waited so long to do it.

Resources

ALTHOUGH your best resources for finding the right doctor are recommendations from people you know, there are also some professional organizations that can be helpful. The following can assist you in your search by providing names of dermatologic surgeons and plastic surgeons in your area who perform liposuction. But remember that when you get these referrals, you are just getting names of qualified members of that organization. You still have to do your research as outlined in this book. These organizations also provide information about liposuction and other cosmetic surgical procedures.

THE AMERICAN SOCIETY FOR DERMATOLOGIC SURGERY
5550 Meadowbrook Drive, Suite 120
Rolling Meadows, IL 60008
Phone: 847-956-0900
Consumer hotline: 1-800-441-2737

Website: www.aboutskinsurgery.com
E-mail: info@aboutskinsurgery.com

THE AMERICAN ACADEMY OF DERMATOLOGY
930 East Woodfield Road
Schaumberg, IL 60173
Phone: 847-330-0230
Websites: www.aad.org and www.skincarephysician.com/
agingskinnet

AMERICAN ACADEMY OF COSMETIC SURGERY
737 North Michigan Avenue, Suite 820
Chicago, IL 60611
Phone: 312-981-6760
Website: www.cosmeticsurgery.org

AMERICAN SOCIETY OF PLASTIC SURGEONS AND PLASTIC
SURGERY EDUCATIONAL FOUNDATION
444 East Algonquin Road
Arlington Heights, IL 60005
Phone: 847-228-9900
Website: www.plasticsurgery.org

AMERICAN SOCIETY FOR AESTHETIC PLASTIC SURGERY
11081 Winner's Circle
Los Alamitos, CA 90720
Phone: 1-800-364-2174
Referral phone line: 1-888-272-7711
Website: www.surgery.org
E-mail: asaps@surgery.org

You can also contact Dr. Shelton's office directly or visit
his website, where you will find information on liposuction
and the many other cosmetic and medical procedures performed in his office.

RON SHELTON, M.D.
THE NEW YORK AESTHETIC CENTER
260 East 66th Street
New York, NY 10021
Phone: 212-593-1818
Fax: 212-832-3990
Website: www.thenyac.com

About the Authors

RON M. SHELTON, M.D., is a board-certified dermatologist and dermatologic surgeon. He studied liposuction during a one-year cosmetic dermatologic surgical fellowship at the University of California, San Francisco, under the mentorship of Dr. Richard Glogau and Dr. Roy Grekin. He was then recruited by the Mount Sinai Medical Center, New York City, to create their first Division of Dermatologic Surgery at Mount Sinai Medical Center in 1993, and remains on the hospital's teaching staff. He has taught liposuction to many local and visiting international physicians through the Mount Sinai cosmetic dermatology fellowship program. He has written articles in medical journals, a textbook chapter on liposuction, and co-authored the book *Botox* (Berkley Books, 2002); and has taught the subject annually at The American Academy of Dermatology conferences for the last several years.

Dr. Shelton was voted one of the Best Doctors in America by Castle-Connolly. His practice entails Mohs micrographic surgery, reconstructive surgery, laser surgery, noninvasive laser rejuvenation, chemical peels, liposuction, fat injections, and Botox and collagen injections. Dr. Shelton has been in private practice since 1998 and is the cofounder of The New York Aesthetic Center, L.L.P. (www.thenyac.com). More information about Dr. Shelton and the multidisciplinary cosmetic surgery practice he and his codirector, Dr. Domenico Valente, have created can be found at the above website or by calling 212-593-1818. They are located at 260 East 66th Street, New York, NY 10021. You may also e-mail them at: thenyac@aol.com.

TERRY MALLOY is a New York–based freelance writer who specializes in health and medical issues. She is the co-author of *Botox* with Dr. Ron Shelton, *Creatine and Other Natural Muscle Boosters* (Dell, 1999), and *Viagra: The Wonder Drug for Peak Performance* (Dell, 1999), and author of *Montessori and Your Child* (Nienhuis, 1992).